AWARENESS HEALS

Awareness Heals

THE FELDENKRAIS METHOD FOR DYNAMIC HEALTH

Steven Shafarman

ADDISON-WESLEY PUBLISHING COMPANY, INC.

Reading, Massachusetts • Menlo Park, California • New York
Don Mills, Ontario • Harlow, England • Amsterdam • Bonn
Sydney • Singapore • Tokyo • Madrid • San Juan
Paris • Seoul • Milan • Mexico City • Taipei

The terms Feldenkrais Method®, Feldenkrais®, Awareness Through Movement®, Functional Integration®, and The Feldenkrais Guild® are Registered Marks of The Feldenkrais Guild®.

Library of Congress Cataloging-in-Publication Data

Shafarman, Steven.
    Awareness heals : the Feldenkrais method for dynamic health /
Steven Shafarman.
      p.   cm.
    Includes bibliographical references and index.
    ISBN 0-201-69469-7
    1. Feldenkrais method.   I. Title.
RC489.F44S53   1997
613.7'1—dc20   96-41924
                                            CIP

Text design and production by Mark Corsey
Interior illustrations by Elizabeth Morales
Cover illustration by Chad Kubo
Set in 10-point New Baskerville

1 2 3 4 5 6 7 8 9–MA–0100999897

First printing, April 1997

Addison-Wesley books are available at special discounts for bulk purchases. For more information about how to make such purchases in the U.S., please contact the Corporate, Government, and Special Sales Department at Addison-Wesley Publishing Company, One Jacob Way, Reading, MA 01867, or call (800) 238-9682.

CONTENTS

To the memory of Moshe Feldenkrais, D.Sc. (1904–1984),
for inspiring and provoking me to learn and think;

For everyone who makes these ideas her or his own—
by doing so you help realize Moshe's dreams.

How to Use This Book

The Feldenkrais Method is both a new approach to movement or exercise and a new way of thinking about health and human behavior. These new ideas may seem quite familiar, however, since the Feldenkrais Method is based on understanding how we learn as babies.

To emphasize the organic quality of the Feldenkrais Method, I designed this book with a symmetrical structure, like your body. In the middle, as the trunk or torso, are six lessons which enable you to experience the Feldenkrais Method and how it reawakens and refines the process through which we learn to move as babies. On each side of the lessons—the book's arms and legs— are three chapters, which relate what and how you are learning to your everyday experience. In extending this analogy, I see this introduction as a hand: I offer it to welcome you to this way of thinking and the benefits of the Feldenkrais Method.

The Method, Moshe, and Me, the first chapter, tells the story of the Feldenkrais Method and its founder, Dr. Moshe Feldenkrais, who I studied with for many years. The second chapter, *The Feldenkrais Method,* shows how you can use the Method generally—and the six lessons in this book in particular—to relieve pain, recover from stress, improve athletic and artistic performance, and enhance pleasure.

The third chapter, *Learning to Learn,* discusses specific ways for you to gain maximum benefit from the six lessons. You will learn and improve most rapidly when you minimize any effort and continually seek to move more comfortably, effectively, and enjoyably. In various ways, reducing excess effort is the essence of this learning, and years of teaching and thousands of students have shown me that most of us tend to work much harder than necessary or desirable. While some readers may want to begin with the lessons, I recommend you read this chapter before doing them. For your convenience, it is quite short.

The six lessons are best learned in the order presented. Each lesson has several parts and often instructs you to pause or rest for a moment. These rests are important for your learning and I encourage you to lie still, breathe easily, and enjoy them. Specific movements are sometimes performed and then repeated; the sequence and repetitions enable you to sense changes and discover differences, which are essential for learning. Lesson Five, *Effortless Sitting*, and Lesson Six, *Elegant Walking*, summarize and integrate movements from the first four lessons. I suggest you allow 45 minutes for each lesson.

You will benefit most from these lessons if you do them on different days to allow time for you to integrate and assimilate. As with learning to play golf or piano, to use a computer or speak a foreign language, reviewing can facilitate learning. After you have done a complete lesson at least once, feel free to skip parts or explore your own variations. Even a few movements can be useful, if you do them with awareness. You may also want to review *Learning to Learn* occasionally.

After the six lessons is another short chapter, *Learning and Life*, which suggests many ways you can integrate learning and the benefits of the lessons into your everyday activities. The final two chapters, *Toward a Science of Health* and *Awareness Heals*, will help you understand the way of thinking that makes the Feldenkrais Method unique and effective. As you will see, these insights into how we learn as babies apply to art, science, medicine, psychology, philosophy, education, and all other aspects of our lives. I conclude the book with *A World of Awareness*, my vision regarding these ideas and what is possible for each of us as individuals and for all of us together.

I encourage you to use this book in whatever way seems to suit you best. Perhaps we'll meet one day and you'll tell me what you learned. If you make these ideas your own, you may discover new ways to apply them that benefit me and many others.

The Method, Moshe, and Me

"My pain's gone."

"I haven't moved so easily in years."

"This way of thinking really makes sense."

"These lessons are so simple and effective, I wish I'd learned them in school."

I hear comments like these every day. The Feldenkrais Method helps people relieve chronic or occasional back pain, shoulder tension, and most other musculoskeletal difficulties. Individuals diagnosed with neurological disorders such as stroke, cerebral palsy, or multiple sclerosis discover easier, healthier ways to function. Artists, athletes, and other performers, both amateurs and world-class professionals, use Feldenkrais lessons to improve their skills.

The basics of the Feldenkrais Method are easy to learn and apply. You can learn each of the simple lessons in this book in less than 45 minutes—and doing them even one time may benefit you for the rest of your life. Whether you are 20, 50, or 80 years old . . . whether you are mostly sedentary, exercise occasionally, or work out in the gym daily . . . whether you are generally healthy or living with some disability . . . these lessons will help you learn to move more comfortably and effectively.

1

Medical doctors, chiropractors, and other health professionals increasingly acknowledge the Feldenkrais Method as a valuable, educational adjunct to their treatments. The Feldenkrais Approach to helping people improve their everyday functioning is quite compatible with the medical focus on treating injuries and illnesses. With many types of therapy, people find that pains or problems recur after a few hours, days, or weeks. Genetics may be blamed, or age or occupation, and people sometimes assume they "just have to learn to live with it." These notions may be unnecessarily limiting and self-fulfilling, however. With the Feldenkrais Method, you can learn to live in ways that minimize or eliminate many problems.

The six lessons in this book use simple, common movements: bending, turning, leaning, breathing, sitting, and walking. When you are more aware and effective with these fundamental skills, you will be better able to do whatever you choose, no matter how complex or demanding.

The Man and His Method

Moshe Feldenkrais had an extraordinary background for his discoveries. Born in the Ukraine in 1904, he left his home and family at the age of 14 to emigrate to Palestine. That was shortly after the end of World War I, and the journey took almost six months, mostly walking. For the next ten years, Feldenkrais lived in Tel Aviv, at that time a relatively small community of pioneering Jewish settlers. As a young man, he studied, worked as a tutor, laborer, and surveyor, and pursued his love of sports. While playing soccer, he tore the ligaments and cartilage in his left knee so severely that his knee was swollen and painful for many months.

Feldenkrais moved to Paris in 1928 to study physics, mathematics, and mechanical and electrical engineering. After earning his Doctor of Science degree at the Sorbonne, he was invited to work with Frédéric Joliot-Curie, director of the Curie Institute, one of the premier scientific laboratories in the world. Joliot-Curie discovered induced radiation and won the 1935 Nobel Prize in Chemistry, and Feldenkrais was Joliot-Curie's principal assistant at the time. Also while in Paris, Feldenkrais met Jigoro Kano, the Japanese Minister of Education and developer of modern judo. Feldenkrais became one of the first Europeans to earn a black belt in judo, founded the Judo Club of Paris, and wrote two books on judo, the first of which included a foreword by Kano in the original French edition.

In 1940, when the Nazis took over Paris, Feldenkrais was on one of the last boats that escaped to England. The people squeezing onto the packed boat were told to leave all their possessions behind, but Feldenkrais refused to abandon a suitcase Joliot-Curie had entrusted to him. That suitcase contained laboratory notes describing research on nuclear fission, plans for an incendiary bomb, and two quarts of heavy water that were later used in the Manhattan Project to build the atomic bomb. Feldenkrais worked for the British Admiralty during World War II, helping to develop sonar and other means of submarine detection. He also continued to practice and teach judo. Throughout those years, he became increasingly interested in human development and how children learn to move, inspired in part by observing babies in the office of his wife, Yona Rubenstein, a pediatrician.

After a bus accident aggravated Feldenkrais's old knee injury, doctors said he needed surgery or he would never again walk normally. This was before the development of modern arthroscopic techniques, and the best surgeons in England offered only a 50-percent chance that an operation would succeed. Feldenkrais thought that performing surgery with such a prognosis was unscientific and irresponsible. As he later recounted, "I told the doctors they had to be idiots, that in my laboratory we would only undertake an experiment when we were 98-percent certain of our hypothesis. Yet they wanted to cut open my knee while admitting that the odds of success were no better than chance." In pursuit of a better answer, he studied everything that was then known about health and healing—anatomy and physiology, neurophysiology, exercise and movement therapies, psychotherapy and spiritual practices, yoga, hypnosis, and acupuncture.

Feldenkrais succeeded in learning to walk again, never had the operation, and even resumed his judo. Through many months of careful, minimal movements with disciplined self-observation, he discovered ways to reawaken and refine the fundamental processes through which young children learn to move and function. The key to healing, he found, is to become more *aware* of what one is doing.

Sometime after Feldenkrais regained full movement in his knee, a friend and fellow scientist who suffered with severe, chronic back pain asked if the same process could help him. It did, and Feldenkrais started to see how these methods might benefit everyone. With one person at a time, he developed ways to facilitate this healing and learning, nonverbally, through touch and movement, and he began to call this *Functional Integration*. Feldenkrais also developed ways to communicate these insights and possibilities to any number of people at the same time by using specific spoken or written directions. This became *Awareness Through Movement*.

In 1950, Feldenkrais returned to Tel Aviv to become the first director of the electronics department of the Israeli Defense Force. Soon after, Feldenkrais was invited to work with Israel's first Prime Minister, David Ben-Gurion, who by then had lived for decades with chronic back pain, breathing difficulties, and other serious problems. Ben-Gurion's health improved dramatically, and Feldenkrais began to be considered a national treasure in Israel. He taught in Israel and Europe through the 1950s and 1960s, and was first invited to the United States in 1971. Feldenkrais returned to the United States many times over the next 11 years, training large groups of practitioners in San Francisco and Amherst, Massachusetts. In 1984, after a series of illnesses, he died peacefully at the age of 80.

I first learned of the Feldenkrais Method in 1974 when I bought his book *Awareness Through Movement* (Harper and Row, 1972). At that time, I was in college and expected to become a teacher or psychologist. I always had been profoundly curious about human behavior and wanted a profession that enabled me to help others while I continued learning.

In the summer of 1975, I studied intensively with Dr. Jean Houston, who has devoted her life to exploring and teaching ways to enhance creativity and other latent capacities. After I graduated from Colby College in June 1976, Jean and her husband, Dr. Robert Masters, invited me to work with them at The Foundation for Mind Research. For me, that was paradise. I was their research associate for the next 18 months, working with Bob on several projects and assisting Jean with her seminars and workshops. While there, I met many extraordinary people, including Margaret Mead, Jean's friend and mentor, who was a regular visitor, and Feldenkrais. Moshe would visit the Foundation whenever he was in New York City, and I enjoyed many hours with him and attended several weekend programs he taught.

Throughout that time, I devoted an hour or more each day to tapes of Awareness Through Movement lessons that Moshe had given to Bob Masters. I benefited significantly from these lessons, feeling taller, lighter, stronger, more agile, better coordinated, and generally healthier. The Feldenkrais Method impressed me as a remarkably effective form of gentle exercise or body-oriented therapy. I was not really interested in the body, however, and decided to continue in psychology to work with the mind. Over the next few years I trained in Ilana Rubenfeld's Synergy Method, learned Neuro-Linguistic Programming, and studied gestalt therapy, Psychosynthesis, and other techniques.

After several years of studying these approaches and using them successfully with many people, I saw Moshe again in the summer of 1980. That was when I began to understand clearly that his insights into health and human behavior were fundamentally different from anything I had been taught. In simple, concrete ways, the Feldenkrais Method eliminates any division between body and mind. I fell in love with his way of thinking.

Nineteen eighty-one was the second year of the Feldenkrais Professional Training Program in Amherst, Massachusetts, and the last time Moshe taught in the United States. Moshe and Jerry Karzen, the organizer of that training, asked me to be Moshe's appointment secretary for the summer. In that capacity I traveled with Moshe, attended a number of his large public workshops, and videotaped many lessons he did with individuals who had been diagnosed with cerebral palsy, multiple sclerosis, and other serious disabilities.

Moshe lived his ideas. He often said that his Method was not a way of teaching or doing therapy, but focused instead on creating conditions for learning. In practice, this meant that in spite of people's expectations, even contrary to what might appear to be his self-interest, Moshe mostly refused to tell people what to do. Being with him presented many challenges for which he provided little or no guidance. While Moshe claimed he did this out of absolute respect for the integrity of each person, his behavior sometimes seemed ridiculous or manipulative. Many people, including some of his longtime students, found him exasperating and intimidating.

I understood why the first time he was annoyed with me. A woman for whom I had been unable to schedule an appointment had managed to get Moshe's private number and called him directly to complain. The following afternoon, in the midst of saying how angry he was that the woman had been upset with me, Moshe abruptly shifted his tone and remarked, "All this time you've been doing a better job with my schedule than anyone ever has. It's been going so smoothly that I keep forgetting to thank you. But now I'm ticked off." Then he began berating me again for not having been more tactful with the woman. Moshe alternately scolded and praised me for several hours, pausing to give lessons when students arrived, resuming for a few minutes between students, and continuing all through dinner. He never allowed me even a moment to present my explanation.

At first I was disturbed and confused, but by the end of the evening I was intrigued and somewhat amused. If Moshe was testing me, as some people later suggested, I must have passed since he was consistently friendly and respectful from then onward. Yet I did not feel as if I was being tested or manipulated; instead, it seemed to me that Moshe was using me and that incident as a catalyst for his own exploring and learning. He seemed as fascinated by his emotional experience and expression as he must have been in discovering the movements that resolved his knee problem.

Through this experience and many others, I began to understand how Moshe's personality was inseparable from his genius. Where most of us crave certainty and want our questions answered immediately, Moshe thrived on doubt and ambiguity, trying to "say yes and no at the same time." He claimed the freedom to discover his own truths and refused to be burdened by anyone's opinions or expectations. At times, Moshe seemed to shift his whole being instantaneously—from a frail, little old man to a powerful young athlete, or from a willful, self-absorbed child to a serene spiritual master. By this eagerness to embody the complete range of his experience, Moshe inspired those of us around him to become more fully and uniquely ourselves. That was the essence of his life and his teaching.

When working with a child who had been diagnosed with cerebral palsy, Down syndrome, or other disorders, Moshe was invariably as sweet and tender as an ideal grandfather. More than that, he insisted that even the youngest child was uniquely aware and intelligent. For this reason, he avoided talking about a child in the child's presence; if he wanted medical information that might involve a negative prognosis, he and the parent would leave the room and talk in the hallway. Children loved him, and many responded in ways that seemed miraculous: I saw a number of children working with Moshe leave their wheelchairs or crutches and walk unassisted for the first time in their lives.

In the years I have practiced the Feldenkrais Method, I have become ever more certain that Moshe's elegant, functional way of thinking is fundamentally true. He sometimes said that his ideas seem terribly complex because they are, in fact, extremely simple. Moshe titled the last book he wrote *The Elusive Obvious* (Meta Publications, 1981) to express his belief that profound truths are often overlooked. Countless people suffer excessively and unnecessarily, in Moshe's view, and common explanations of human behavior frequently obscure more than they enlighten.

I first read *The Elusive Obvious* as a photocopied manuscript while sitting next to Moshe on an airplane. As I finished each chapter, he put his hand on the pages to prevent me from reading further while he asked me what I thought. The game, I realized immediately, was to praise the book in a different way at each interruption. At one point I said, "You know, Moshe, while reading this I feel that the hopes and dreams I had as a child are still valid, and that society was wrong to tell me otherwise." He grinned from ear to ear. In that book and everything he did, his intention was to inspire people to trust their experience, think for themselves, and pursue their dreams.

Mastering the Method

For more than 12 years, I have dedicated myself to refining what I learned with Moshe. As my skill with the Method grew, I became increasingly frustrated, sad at times, and even angry that these remarkably simple and powerful ideas were not generally known. This book emerged from my desire to identify a few fundamental lessons and present the thinking that makes them so effective. I have taught the following six lessons to children in school, adults at their jobs, and residents of convalescent homes in wheelchairs. Thousands of people have convinced me through their experiences that these lessons can provide significant, lasting benefits to everyone who learns them.

Some of the stories I tell may sound dramatic, yet most of my colleagues report similar successes. Contrary to the claims of many of my students, I do not believe I have any special power to heal. Rather, I see the Feldenkrais Method as fundamentally educational, a way for you or anyone else to learn to move more comfortably and effectively. You benefit from increasing awareness, from what you learn about yourself, not from what I say or do. In this way, the Method can evoke the capacity for healing and health within each and every individual. Moshe acknowledged that even though his methods might appear magical or miraculous, they are actually simple and scientific—and can be learned by anyone.

Every person I have worked with has taught me in a different way that all pains and problems involve lack of awareness. I hope and expect that these six lessons and the thinking they present will do more than teach you how to relieve pain, recover from stress, and enhance pleasure. In whatever you do, the Feldenkrais Method can help you become more aware, comfortable, effective, and healthy.

The Feldenkrais Method

We commonly say that children learn to walk and talk, but rarely consider how that learning occurs. Children learn by exploring and imitating, guided by comfort and motivated by curiosity. In most cases, however, people cease to explore a task once they attain a minimal level of competence at it. Furthermore, each of the parents, teachers, peers, and media figures we imitate displays a complex mix of abilities and inabilities, good habits and bad ones. In exploring and imitating, knowingly and unknowingly, each of us acquires some poor habits with no memory of how we learned them or what alternatives might be possible.

Back pain is an example of a common problem that is often related to bad habits. For many people, back pain is chronic and costly. Treatments typically identify some specific cause—muscles too weak or too tense, the spine misaligned, or nerves pinched—and then try to correct the problem with drugs or surgery, exercises or manipulations, psychotherapy or relaxation techniques. Numerous techniques can provide relief, at least temporarily. For lasting benefits, however, people need to learn more efficient ways of moving. When you move comfortably and effectively, muscles will contract only when necessary while remaining loose at all other times, and the spine will continually align and realign appropriately for whatever you are doing.

Each of us acts in accordance with how we sense and think about ourselves, a self-image which forms and changes with learning and experience. A complete self-image would include continuous awareness of every joint in the skeleton and the entire surface of the skin, functioning dynamically in every act. In contrast with this ideal, many people view the body as a collection of separate, independently moving parts: feet, legs, hands, arms, head, and a lump in the middle that holds everything together.

To appreciate how everyone's self-image has some gaps and inaccuracies, consider what occurs with limping: Almost everyone has stubbed a toe or sprained an ankle at some time, most of us more than once, so you know what it means to alter your way of walking in order to reduce pressure on an injured foot. Yet you have probably never thought about what a complicated activity limping is. Recall, if you can, a time when you had to limp. If you like, put this book down and re-create that experience, or at least imagine doing so. Stand and try to walk so that the little toe of one foot remains completely off the floor, as if any movement or contact there were painful. Sense how you do that, the various efforts involved. That is quite different from your normal way of walking, I hope and expect.

You limp as a whole person, not with your foot only. The ankle and knee of the affected leg stiffen while the opposite leg compensates, your pelvis and both hip joints twist asymmetrically, and those imbalances involve your back and neck, how you swing your arms, and how you turn your head. All of these changes occur instantly, spontaneously, without thought or preparation, and, most of the time, without awareness. In adapting to something as seemingly inconsequential as a stubbed little toe, you alter how you move everywhere. Then, soon after the toe heals, again mostly without awareness or intention, you stop limping and resume walking normally. You stop limping in the same way and for the same reason that you learned to walk initially— walking is quicker and easier than limping or crawling.

You may not have stopped limping completely, however. There may be some lingering imbalance or disturbance, some slightly increased tension in a few muscles, in your back, shoulders, or hip joints. While someone with an ideal self-image would be aware of subtle changes, for most of us such changes would be ignored or overlooked. Yet even one-hundredth of one percent of unnecessary effort, multiplied by the thousands of movements each of us makes every day, can lead to significant problems after a few years. Inefficiencies of this sort may explain chronic pain, fibromyalgia, repetitive strain disorders, and many other problems. With arthritis, for example, calcium deposits in the joints may be natural ways of protecting and reinforcing tissues from the subtle stresses of inefficient movements.

All but the most delicate movements of the eyes, face, or hands require you to shift some weight and adjust large muscles in your trunk. Your brain constantly monitors input from all sensory receptors, every muscle, each joint in the skeleton, the entire surface of the skin, and all internal organs. From this neurological perspective, your whole being actively engages in everything you do all the time, even when you think you are doing nothing. The only way a part of you can be left out of an act is to leave that part in bed when you get up in the morning. In all that you do, you act as a complete person. Ignoring or neglecting yourself, even partially, impairs your ability to do what you want.

When I talk to people about these ideas, almost everyone responds at some point by saying, "This makes sense." Yet I do not want you to accept anything I say simply because you like the idea, or because you see me as some kind of authority, or for any other abstract reason. The lessons in this book are designed to enable you to test these ideas for yourself. Real learning, in my opinion, requires direct experience.

One way to appreciate how every movement involves all of yourself is to sense how you lift your head. Now, or at the next convenient opportunity, lie on your back with your arms at your sides. You can lie on the floor or on a bed, although a firmer surface will provide more accurate feedback. Lift and lower your head, simply, slowly, easily, several times. Make a small movement, just an inch or so. Use as little effort as possible. Observe what you do when you lift and lower your head. If you really want to learn—please, stop reading and do this.

You can certainly sense the effort in your neck muscles as you lift your head. Your head weighs 12 to 16 pounds, like a bowling ball.

Perhaps you also notice some activity in your chest and upper back. Rest for a moment so that you do not fatigue those muscles; making a small, slow movement like this involves more effort than most of us realize.

Now place your hands on your lower abdomen, with your fingertips touching your pubic bone at the base of your pelvis. Rest your hands lightly to sense the muscles there with your fingers. Lift your head and lower it a few more times. Do you perceive the muscular effort in your lower abdomen? If that is not clear, hold your head in the air for a few moments. Sense how the muscles at the pubic bone release when you lower your head. By the way, did you hold your breath while doing that?

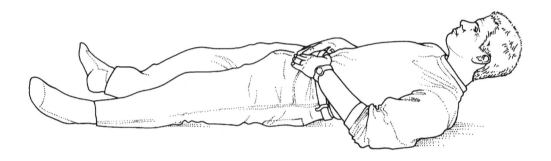

After sensing that muscles at your pubic bone were working with those in your neck to lift or lower your head, you might acknowledge that muscles were working throughout your chest and abdomen also. The first time you did this, you probably were not aware of the fact that lifting your head involves muscular efforts throughout your trunk, front and back, and into your pelvis and hip joints. Rest for another moment and sense the movement in your chest and abdomen as you breathe. Now, breathing easily and more aware, lift and lower your head again once or twice. Do you notice any change from when you first did this? Most people find that they lift their head higher, with less effort.

As this simple experience shows, enhancing awareness increases strength and skill, spontaneously.

Awareness and Learning

Feldenkrais lessons are extremely pleasant and relaxing, yet this is more of an added benefit than a goal. Whether I am seeing an individual or teaching a class, I want to stimulate a learning process so that people continue to improve on their own. The six lessons in this book have helped me to do that with many of my students.

One such student was Marcy, who had been having migraine headaches, occasionally several in a week, for almost 20 years. At times, these were so severe that she went to the emergency room for an injection of pain medication. A variety of treatments had helped, and Marcy had been in a hospital-based program for people with chronic pain that included psychotherapy, stress management, biofeedback, physical therapy, exercise, and relaxation techniques. Doctors had told Marcy she no longer had true migraines, only cluster headaches, yet she still suffered, both from headaches and from side effects of the drugs. In spite of this, at age 35 Marcy was completing her Ph.D. in mathematics.

Marcy almost always arrived at my office with a headache, her face dark and drawn inward, eyes shaded and lips pressed tightly together. She left each lesson smiling and free from pain. When I asked Marcy how the headaches began, she said she just did not know. She would feel fine when she sat down to study, but three or four hours later pain would force her to stop. In response to my questions, Marcy realized that she concentrated so totally on what was in front of her that she was not at all aware of how she was sitting, or even if she was breathing. I talk with many people who experience chronic or persistent problems, and most of them acknowledge a similar lack of awareness.

When I see a student individually, I usually ask the person to remove his or her shoes and lie, fully clothed, on a low padded table. Then, sitting on a stool next to the table, I gently turn the person's head, lift an arm or leg, and generally explore the pattern of movement everywhere. I proceed carefully, guided by my sense of what the person feels and needs at each moment, so that he or she is always comfortable. Through specific sequences and precise movements, I evoke the process by which babies learn to crawl and walk, shaping that process to the student's unique needs at that particular moment. Just as babies outgrow crawling when they learn to walk, my students, over time, replace old habits and tensions with new awareness and skill.

Marcy improved from the first lesson. She had trouble, however, learning to integrate these new skills into her everyday activities; her habit of concentrating was just too intense, her neglect of herself too complete. We had to develop specific signals that would tell Marcy to pause, breathe, and recall the lessons and how she was learning to move comfortably. For a while, Marcy set a timer to remind her periodically to stop working. That was effective, yet I did not want to leave her dependent on external cues. In our final lessons, I helped Marcy become aware of moving her arms to turn the pages of the book she was studying, and she was able to begin using that as a cue to alter her position and to breathe more fully.

I saw Marcy only 15 times before she moved to another city. When I last spoke with her, more than one year after our final lesson, Marcy reported that her headaches were no longer a significant problem. She said that at times she would fall back into her habit of concentrating too intensely, but usually at the first sign of a headache she was able to relieve it by applying what she had learned. When she did have a headache it was less severe and resolved more quickly, almost always without medication. Marcy also told me that her work was going well, and that the lessons had helped her become more aware and skillful in many activities in addition to studying.

Conventional approaches define migraine headaches as a pain to be relieved or a problem to be treated. I see them from a completely different perspective, and to me Marcy's headaches seemed to be the only way she knew to escape the rigidity of her acquired habits of straining, stiffening, and holding her breath. Instead of trying to treat or relieve her migraines, I helped her learn to be more aware and comfortable. Relief from pain was her reward for enhancing awareness.

Whether someone comes to me for some minor stress or discomfort, or after being diagnosed with a neurological disorder as severe as stroke or multiple sclerosis, I look at the specific ways he or she moves. The Feldenkrais Method works with the person, not with the symptom or disease. Whatever someone's history or the apparent cause of a problem may be, I focus on helping each individual learn how to be better today and tomorrow. To improve, the first step is to be aware of how one functions at this moment, here/now.

As you read this, you may be sitting, lying in bed, or standing, perhaps in a bookstore. Pause and notice how you are and what you are doing. Simply observe yourself for a moment. Do you sense where you contact the chair, the bed, or the ground? Are you aware of the position and weight of your pelvis, your back, and your head? Does your head contact a chair, a pillow, or only space? What about your arms as you hold this book, and your legs—where are your limbs relative to your trunk?

Of course, you can be aware when you want to be. Most of the time, however, each of us acts in habitual ways with only limited awareness of how we are moving and what we are doing. Are you comfortable? Or are you in some habitual posture which actually feels somewhat awkward when you pause to observe yourself?

Now, notice something more: without thinking about it, without trying, simply in the process of becoming aware, you have almost certainly altered your position slightly to increase your comfort. We do that spontaneously when we sense any strain, stiffness, or fatigue.

Awareness heals.

Relieve Pain

According to medical science, pain may be caused by an irritation or blockage of nerve fibers, too much or too little blood pressure due to a disruption in circulation, a buildup of lactic acid or other waste products in the tissues, or some combination of these and other factors. One does not need a doctor or scientist, however, to know that whatever the cause, pain occurs when something is wrong. Pain indicates a deviation from normal, acceptable, functioning.

Yet pain is essential to life. Children born without the ability to experience pain, a rare and serious neurological defect, survive only through the constant vigilance of their parents and care-takers. Without pain, they have no way to avoid injury, cutting themselves, biting their fingers, even poking out their own eyes. Pain is a necessary guide in learning about ourselves and our world.

Each of us responds to pain by avoiding any movements that might hurt. This is innate; all mammals do the same. This response is generally useful and healthy for a limited time, but continued immobility prevents healing.

Carolyn came to me after several doctors and dentists had told her that her neck pain, headaches, and jaw problems were caused by temporomandibular joint syndrome, TMJ. One dentist had recommended surgery to correct an imbalance in the joint. Another told Carolyn that an operation would not be necessary if she avoided opening her mouth too widely and ate only soft foods that did not require much chewing. When I saw her, Carolyn had been doing that for several years.

After listening to this story, I asked Carolyn, "How can you possibly learn to move more easily if you continue to avoid many movements? Just because something was painful in the past, doesn't mean it will always be difficult." After only two lessons, Carolyn was able to open her mouth freely. Her headaches disappeared, she could move her neck and shoulders more comfortably, and she was again able to enjoy apples and corn-on-the-cob, which had been among her favorite foods. Carolyn came to see me several weeks after the lessons and happily reported that she had begun writing poetry again, after not having done so for a few years, and that she had resolved some problems in her marriage. She credited these breakthroughs to the way I had helped her learn to move more comfortably.

Instead of interpreting pain as a signal to avoid movement, we can allow pain to guide us to learn to act more skillfully. Pain can be a most effective teacher, if we are aware and know how to learn.

Where movement is restricted, muscles become weak, joints calcify, circulation is reduced, and, Moshe realized, areas of the nervous system are continually inhibited. Healthy children fall down and bounce back, spontaneously letting go of fixed patterns and moving on to discover new possibilities. As we age, however, we become, literally, set in our ways.

Many people with pain in one hand or hip joint or shoulder believe the cause is arthritis, and I have heard doctors say that everyone over 35 has signs of this disease. When I have asked doctors about this, however, not one has been able to explain why age might bring the problem in a particular joint or on only one side, since the other side and joints are just as old. Physical limitations are commonly viewed as inevitable aspects of aging, yet habits and lack of awareness play a significant role. Furthermore, the belief that age or arthritis is the cause of problems often leads people to restrict activities, which may contribute to further stiffness and other difficulties. Elderly people can certainly move quite skillfully; Moshe was 77 when I was traveling with him, and he still enjoyed demonstrating judo. I have helped many people diagnosed with arthritis to improve significantly, often dramatically, by becoming more aware and learning to move more efficiently. When I was young, my mother would dismiss my occasional complaints of stiffness or discomfort as "growing pains," and I now believe that one can have growing pains and keep learning at any age.

People experiencing severe pain typically orient every act around the pain, frequently thinking about how to avoid or reduce discomfort. In doing that, however, they continually reinforce the idea that something is wrong. My first goal with someone in such situations is to find a movement the person can do comfortably, no matter how small or subtle the movement might be. I may spend a whole lesson exploring a pleasant gesture with the hand or simple shifting of the eyes. This often brings dramatic benefits. As people learn to be more aware and move in ways that feel good, at least relatively, the pattern of pain and immobility is broken and healing becomes possible.

When people are experiencing pain, they often have difficulty sleeping. Typically, people look for some comfortable position and then try to remain still, waiting to fall asleep, and often worrying that they will not be able to do so. Stillness often leads to stiffness, however, when one is unaware. I teach people to do simple, easy movements instead. You can do the lessons in this book so gently that you are not sure if you are actually moving or only dreaming about moving. Some of my students have described this as "rocking myself to sleep," and those who try this say it is so restful they no longer worry about sleeping. People also report waking up feeling much more refreshed, without any customary stiffness or discomfort. A number of my students have told me that they quit using sleeping pills once they began doing the lessons in this book.

This demonstrates a fundamental truth of the Feldenkrais Method: Awareness and attitude are more important than any specific act. It is not what we do that matters, but how. This applies to all of life.

Recover from Stress

Stress seems to cause certain illnesses and to make most pains or problems worse. Many people talk about how we need to avoid, control, manage, or reduce stress. Yet stress is not an object, a thing of some kind that can be manipulated in these ways. Furthermore, stress is often unavoidable: Accidents happen. Too many demands can be put upon too little time. People quarrel, become ill, die.

Moshe saw that trying to control or manage stress often limits choices and inhibits spontaneity. He spoke of recovering from stress instead, and saw the capacity to do so as a key aspect of health and vitality. I find that emphasizing recovery encourages one to learn, explore, and discover new possibilities. Whenever you experience stress, whatever you may identify as the cause, source, or reason, you will recover more quickly and completely when you are aware of how you are moving or not moving.

Recall an incident when you experienced significant stress. Recall where you were and what was happening. Now contrast that with some time when you felt especially comfortable and confident. You might do that by simply picturing yourself in the two different situations, one stressful and one pleasant. To facilitate your awareness and learning, if you like, you may want to reenact those incidents to help identify the differences. What, specifically, did you sense each time? Compare the movement of your head and shoulders, the way you were sitting, standing, breathing, and relating to other people or the environment. The more vividly you make this comparison, the more you will learn about your behaviors and attitudes.

By observing yourself in these ways and reflecting on your experience, you may find that whenever you feel stress, whatever the apparent cause, your breathing is disturbed. The experience of stress always involves altering the rate and rhythm of breathing, with corresponding changes in movement and muscle tone in the chest, neck, and shoulders. While breathing is partially innate, we also learn to breathe, and to restrict breathing, through the same process by which all movement is learned. Lesson Four, *Uninhibited Breathing*, will help you become more aware of what you are doing while breathing. Then you will be able to breathe more freely, even under conditions that have been stressful in the past.

I have seen a number of people who had been prescribed some medication because of stress, anxiety, or depression. Every one of these people held various muscles extremely tight, with habitually shallow breathing and restricted movement. Medication may help someone cope and be useful for a limited time, but drugs also reduce one's sensitivity and ability to learn.

When I talk to psychiatrists and other doctors, I sometimes ask them deliberately to stiffen and breathe shallowly so they can appreciate what their patients might be feeling. After they do that for a few moments, I tell them, "You would be stressed, anxious, or depressed, too, if you habitually breathed that way." Before I understood the Feldenkrais Method, I thought I could do something to help the mind while ignoring the body, so I am not surprised that most psychiatrists and psychologists are unaware of how their patients are sitting and breathing. We are all relatively alienated from our immediate sensory-motor experience. Among the doctors I know, the majority are relatively stiff, shallow breathers, and surveys show that doctors have higher than average rates of depression and emotional problems.

In learning to breathe more freely, you will discover ways to become more comfortable any time you experience stress or tension. Breathing more easily will help you prevent or relieve stress-related or psychosomatic disorders, including migraine headaches, ulcers, back pain, and many other difficulties. Whatever you normally do or have done in the past, you can learn to act more effectively, even under adverse, stressful conditions. In many cases, you will act so skillfully and spontaneously that unnecessary stresses and unhealthy responses simply cease to occur.

Instead of trying to avoid, control, manage, or reduce stress, we can learn. Any time you experience stress, you can use that as a reminder to breathe and move more comfortably and effectively. In this way, stress can motivate us to make a better life for ourselves, for those we love, and for our whole society and planet.

Improve Athletic and Artistic Performance

My students often want to know what kind of exercise they should do or avoid doing. I generally respond by asking, "What do you enjoy?" Whether you jog, play golf, practice yoga, take aerobics classes, or use high-tech exercise machines, you are more likely to be attentive to your own comfort while doing what pleases you. In addition, when you do what you enjoy and enjoy what you do, you are usually motivated to increase your skill and awareness.

Almost everyone feels better with exercise, and people have many additional reasons for doing it: they have been told that exercise is good for them; they are worried about high blood pressure or cholesterol; or they want to achieve the tight, hard look they see modeled in magazines and on television. Yet I have known many people who hurt themselves while exercising, even under the supervision of a trainer or therapist. It seems to me the likelihood of injury increases anytime an activity is done for some goal other than immediate enjoyment. While self-discipline and willpower are desirable, people sometimes have an attitude of "no pain, no gain," and I view this as a prescription for suffering. "Where there is too much will," Moshe used to say, "there is no skill."

The goal in most systems of exercise is to stretch or strengthen muscles, to do more repetitions, or to work out for a longer period. Comfort is rarely considered. The Feldenkrais Method demonstrates how increasing awareness eliminates excess effort and tensions that interfere with performance. When you learn to be more aware and skillful, you naturally develop speed, strength, and flexibility. Any kind of training or practice becomes more productive and enjoyable.

In the summer of 1981, Julius "Dr. J" Erving, the great basketball player, came for several lessons with Moshe. Dr. J was bent over and limping slightly, with an injured ankle that was not improving. After giving him a lesson one afternoon, Moshe went to watch Dr. J play an exhibition game. The next day, Moshe spoke about how magnificently Dr. J moved on the court. While running and dribbling the ball, Dr. J was able to turn his head freely from side to side so that he could constantly observe the other players and the basket.

Like Dr. J, successful performers in every sport or activity display a well-developed awareness and ability to move efficiently. That is an important key to their success. From the tips of the toes and fingers to the top of the head, every muscle contracts only as needed at each moment, with no wasted effort. This quality of movement is beautiful to see, which is one reason most of us enjoy watching great athletes. People's learning, however, is often limited to specific contexts. Someone might move magnificently while playing basketball or doing yoga, but remain stiff and clumsy at other times. Off the court, Dr. J was not nearly as aware and skillful as on it. As a Feldenkrais practitioner, I am interested in how people move during their *everyday* activities.

Awareness is more important than genetic endowment or training. There have been many great athletes whose bodies were far from ideal, while others who seem to have the perfect physique for a particular sport never achieve success. Training without awareness often has a negative effect, since practice strengthens bad habits and overworks already tight muscles. Mindless repetition, whether on the basketball court, at the piano, or on a factory assembly line, reduces awareness.

Research has demonstrated the value of visualization techniques for improving performance, and a number of books have taught the "inner game" and similar practices. These approaches, however, often overlook the fact that imagining and visualizing involve subtle skills which we acquire only after we have learned to move in more basic ways. Someone who is relatively unaware will often visualize inaccurately, in which case these techniques will provide only minimal benefits. Lesson Three, *Leaning and Lifting*, demonstrates how the Feldenkrais Method relates movement and visualization to enhance both skills.

Sandra, a professional musician, came to see me after pain in the wrists and hands, diagnosed as carpal tunnel syndrome, had forced her to stop performing. I helped her sense how moving her hands involved her arms, shoulders, back, legs, and everywhere else. After a few individual lessons and a class with the six lessons in this book, Sandra told me she was rediscovering the delight she experienced when she began playing clarinet at the age of eight. That enjoyment, she and I agreed, was more valuable than merely relieving her pain. Since her Feldenkrais lessons, Sandra has been performing regularly, and she says that she continues to learn in many ways, increasing both her enjoyment and her skill. Her awareness, I am certain, also makes her an exceptional teacher.

A number of famous musicians and other artists, including violinist Yehudi Menuhin, classical guitarist Narciso Yepes, and theater director Peter Brook, were Moshe's friends and students. Moshe believed that the greatest performers in any field are those who pursue their activity as a path toward greater awareness, not just to please the crowd or for the money. This attitude seems to be what separates the best from all others.

A person can play the piano while focusing on the keys, the fingers, or the notes written on the sheet music. In the process, the musician may hold his or her breath, tighten the shoulders and arms, and ignore the neck, back, and pelvis. Discomfort and fatigue frequently accompany this kind of practice, and many performers live with almost constant pain. In contrast, really playing music involves one's whole being—every cell and muscle fiber, one's total experience with the instrument, the piece, and life, all in harmony.

Many athletes and artists, amateurs and professionals, have told me they wish their early instruction had focused on awareness, rather than achievement or technique. Anyone, by learning to be more aware, can discover new talents and abilities. Each of us can be a gifted amateur, experiencing real skill and satisfaction in many areas.

Dedicated artists and athletes devote a great deal of time to their activity as they continue to refine their skill and understanding. One might have a similar attitude toward the activities of daily life. Sitting in a car or at a computer might be approached with the same awareness as sitting at a piano on stage at Carnegie Hall. You can be as fully alive and present walking into the supermarket as you would be running in the Olympics. As we learn to value ourselves and our everyday experience more fully, we help make life more enjoyable for ourselves and everyone else.

Enhance Pleasure

Most of us are concerned about health and appearance, yet we usually ignore how we are moving, except when something hurts. To me, that attitude—pain or nothing—seems rather sad and limiting. Instead of being satisfied at the mere absence of pain, you can enjoy an ongoing sense of physical pleasure in your everyday experience, the way you breathe, sit, and walk.

This belief is based on Moshe's comments and on my own experience since I began with the Feldenkrais Method. For confirmation, however, I look to a much more reliable source—observing and interacting with some of the wisest and most aware members of our species: babies. A sense of pleasure guides all learning in early childhood. Every baby knows that putting the fingers in the mouth can be ecstasy, lifting the head an exquisite joy, playing with the toes a timeless source of pure delight. When we were young children, each of us was exquisitely attuned to our own comfort, and this awareness informed every act.

My students sometimes ask what caused their problems or how their difficulties might have begun. I like to respond with my own question, "When did you stop skipping?" Young children spontaneously run and skip and dance, and they prefer that to walking in a straight line at a measured pace. Children play. Babies learn to crawl and walk as part of the process of expressing curiosity and making sense of the world. Through that process, they acquire the strength and skill for ever greater efforts. Babies do not do sit-ups, yet for their size and weight, babies and children are much stronger than adults.

Most of what we call education is really socialization. Each of us was taught to act in predictable, socially approved ways. We learned to sit still when we wanted to run and play, to whisper when we wanted to sing and shout, to stiffen our chests and restrict our breathing while ignoring or denying our feelings.

You can learn to move more freely and spontaneously, regardless of your age or any previous illnesses or injuries. A general experience of pleasure can be the background to whatever you do, as it was when you were a child. It is not necessary to be young and supple, because pleasure and pain are always relative. You will begin to feel greater comfort with even a slight improvement from your present condition, and you will realize increasing pleasure as you continue to refine your abilities.

Lesson Six, *Elegant Walking*, will help you sense a comfortable motion in your pelvis as you shift your weight with every step. As this feeling of grace and fluidity becomes normal and natural, you will discover that walking can help you eliminate stiffness or unnecessary effort anywhere. In addition, increasing your ease and comfort while walking will enhance your skill in running, dancing, skiing, tennis, and all related activities.

One activity which almost everyone associates with pleasure is sex. Sex is not just a matter of lips, breasts, genitals, or other "erogenous zones," although people sometimes talk about sex as if that were the case. Sexual activity involves sensation and movement everywhere, indeed, everywhere in both partners. While many books and people describe sex, I have not found anyone who speaks as concretely as Moshe did about the importance of awareness and skillful movement for sexual pleasure. As an example, Moshe observed that people with any sexual dysfunction, such as frigidity or premature ejaculation, always exhibit some general limitation in mobility of the hip joints and pelvis. He also identified improvement in the range and quality of movement in people who were "cured" of their problems, regardless of how that "cure" came about. Do you know how your hip joints and pelvis move during sexual intercourse?

In 1977, I attended a workshop Moshe was teaching in New York City. When working with large groups, more than 300 on this occasion, Moshe would talk to the participants near him as a way to engage everyone who was present. Moshe taught a lesson that weekend on increasing the mobility of the pelvis, a version of which is included in this book as Lesson Five, *Effortless Sitting*. In the front row was a man in his late forties or early fifties who was having difficulty, so Moshe guided him through the first part of the lesson in some detail. The muscles in this man's abdomen and hip joints were very tight, and he said that he used to do sit-ups regularly. The lesson continued, and about 20 minutes after speaking with Moshe the man was moving his pelvis freely, with his hips, chest, and spine coordinating nicely. Upon noticing this, Moshe declared, "Your wife should pay me extra for teaching you this." The man laughed, along with most of the people in the room.

Where you move easily you feel light and alive, and anyone touching you will readily sense that. Whether from a casual pat on the back or a prolonged, intimate caress, each of us can recognize a different quality in the touch of one person or another. Most of us prefer to touch and be touched by someone who is aware and gentle. Hugging a person whose chest is hard and rigid is not nearly as nice as hugging someone who is supple, where the ribs and chest move freely and melt against you. Of course, even the stiffest bodies soften and merge when people really love one another.

As you become more aware and learn to move with greater skill, you will discover many ways to enhance pleasure—for yourself and everyone you touch.

Learning to Learn

The Feldenkrais Method involves learning, and learning is different from training, practicing, or exercising. You will benefit most from the lessons in this book when you clearly understand these differences.

In various ways, conventional approaches to exercise discourage learning and awareness: Mirrors and sexy outfits distract attention. Repetition reinforces existing habits. Music, whether driving rock or Haydn or Bach, dictates a particular pace. Goal-setting, record-keeping, or otherwise focusing on achievements imposes an objective orientation.

To learn and become more aware, with Awareness Through Movement lessons and generally, you want to be present and attentive to your changing experience at each moment.

We learn most easily when comfortable. Before you begin each of the following lessons, especially the first time you do a lesson, take an extra moment to prepare and insure your comfort. Notice what you are wearing, the light and temperature of the room, the space where you will be lying or sitting. While we can ignore distractions, and in our everyday activities we often need to, you will gain the most benefit from these lessons when you do what you can to arrange comfortable conditions.

Do each movement with minimal effort, since excess effort leads to fatigue and interferes with sensing. Each time you repeat a movement, see if you can reduce your effort and move more easily. Always do less than you can. To sense a movement clearly, you may need to repeat it 15 or 20 times. Those final movements may be so subtle that you cannot tell whether you are doing the movement or only imagining it.

An excellent way to do the lessons is to alter your focus frequently. From moment to moment, you can redirect your attention to a different area, joint, or muscle, or to your overall sense and image of yourself. By actively shifting your attention among the details and to the big picture, you will continually enhance your awareness and fill in gaps in your self-image. This is essential, since whatever we do habitually always seems normal and correct. By reducing your efforts and shifting your focus, you identify habits, how they function and are maintained, while simultaneously learning and discovering more desirable alternatives.

The instructions will sometimes ask you to sense distinctions between different movements. At first, some of these distinctions may seem rather subtle or elusive. If you continue to reduce your effort, you will soon find them simple and obvious. In the chapter *Toward a Science of Health,* I explain the scientific, neurological reasons why becoming more aware and eliminating excessive efforts is essential for making precise and accurate distinctions.

As you do these lessons, cultivate an attitude of exploring, discovering, and experimenting. You may find it helpful to imagine yourself as a baby or young child. At the same time, however, you will gain the greatest benefit by following the sequence and not doing extraneous movements. While playing and moving randomly is fun and can be extremely beneficial, people commonly do so in relatively habitual ways. Each sequence is carefully designed to promote learning.

To do these lessons, all you need is space to lie down and a good chair. Lesson Six, *Elegant Walking,* also involves standing and walking around. If you lie on a mat, pad, or rug, it should not be uneven or overly soft because that will interfere with your ability to sense accurately. For the same reason, a simple stool or wooden chair, like many kitchen chairs, is preferable to anything more cushioned. A chair without arms will afford greater mobility than one that has them.

Some more specific hints and suggestions:

- Set aside time when you will not be disturbed.

- A good time to do the lessons is before going to bed, when you are relatively relaxed. You may then want to recall the sensations before you rise in the morning.

- Wear loose, comfortable clothes. Tight jeans may seem comfortable, yet they often restrict mobility of hip joints and pelvis.

- If your attention wanders at any time, pause. Continue only when you are again present. If you fall asleep for a moment, simply resume the lesson when you awaken.

- Always move within your range of ease and comfort. If you begin with small, slow, simple movements, you will discover that larger and more powerful actions can be almost effortless.

- If you sense any pain or discomfort, anywhere, at any time during the lesson, stop. Make the movement smaller, slower, simpler, or in your imagination only. Adjust your position if necessary, even if that means modifying the instructions.

- Do not try to do any movement "well" or according to any specific idea of how it should be or look. If something seems awkward or sloppy, a useful way to learn is deliberately to make it worse.

- The drawings that accompany these lessons are meant to help you interpret the instructions, not to show how *you* should look when you do the movements. Be aware of what you sense, not concerned with your appearance.

- When the instruction is to rest, do so simply. Stretching, wiggling, or otherwise moving around interferes with sensing differences and learning new possibilities.

- Above all, enjoy yourself. More than learning any specific movements or lessons, you are learning to learn. And learning, as every healthy child knows, is great fun.

- After the lesson, allow some time to reflect on your experience and observe any differences, instead of rushing into some activity. Later, or the next day, occasionally recall the movements and perhaps review one or two. See if you can discover ways that these movements relate to everyday activities.

A final suggestion: Many people who begin Awareness Through Movement lessons discover that they frequently stiffen or hold their breath for no apparent reason, during the lessons or while engaging in their usual activities. This can be quite disturbing, and my students sometimes express frustration and doubts about their ability to learn and improve. Most of us are quick to feel bad, to blame ourselves for doing what we think is wrong. Yet we all hold our breath when we feel uncomfortable or anxious, or sometimes simply from habit.

In the past, you were almost certainly holding your breath at least as often as now, but you were not aware of doing so. From now on, any time you sense straining or holding of your breath, congratulate yourself. You are becoming more aware. You will soon discover that you have spontaneously started to breathe and move more freely, even under circumstances in which you had previously stressed and held your breath.

Trust yourself and your learning process, and enjoy.

Bending and Breathing

Lower back pain and stiff necks—we often talk about these common problems while remaining generally much less aware of the mid-back. Furthermore, people typically view these two areas as separate, and most treatments focus only on specific places that are painful. Yet among the thousands of people with neck or lower back pain who have come to see me, every one has also had restricted mobility in the mid-back. It seems to me that trying to help the neck or lower back while ignoring the whole spine is illogical and unlikely to provide more than temporary relief. Whenever muscles are tight or painful in one area, movement everywhere will be disturbed and inefficient.

This lesson will teach you to move your entire spine more freely and harmoniously. When you are aware and do that, you will be able to relieve and often eliminate pain or stiffness anywhere.

In 1985, one year after I moved to Santa Barbara, a professional dancer came to see me because of severe, constant lower back pain. Sylvia had already been to several doctors, and had tried physical therapy, chiropractic, and various exercise techniques, without much benefit. A number of people had advised her to stop dancing, which she did not want to do. When describing her pain, Sylvia said she felt as if she was "leaving a trail of powdered bone wherever I go."

Sylvia had been told to do sit-ups to strengthen her abdominal muscles. This exercise is often recommended for people with lower back pain. Sit-ups may help some people, yet they seem to harm others, and in Sylvia's case that advice was clearly inappropriate. As a teenager, Sylvia had been the sit-up champion at her high school, able to outdo any of the boys, and many afternoons she would go home from school and do 300 or more for practice. Her abdominal muscles were already strong, and with her dancing, she exercised more than most people. What Sylvia needed was to learn to move and breathe more comfortably and efficiently. None of the doctors or therapists had taught her how to do that, or even mentioned it.

In a number of individual lessons and a few classes, I helped Sylvia learn the Bending and Breathing patterns in this lesson and other ways to move more easily. Two years after seeing me, Sylvia was dancing in Santa Barbara's annual Summer Solstice parade, a two-hour festival along State Street. When she saw me standing among the spectators, I waved, and she yelled out, "Thanks for fixing me." Sylvia is still dancing, now ten years later. When I told her that I was going to use her story in my book, she thanked me again and said she regularly reviews those few lessons and continues to benefit.

Remember to keep each movement small and easy, within the range of complete comfort. If you have problems with your neck or lower back, be especially careful. Do only minimal movements in any area that is or has been painful, while looking for ways to move more freely everywhere else. I have taught this lesson to people diagnosed with herniated disks in their necks or lower backs, some of whom had refused surgery and others of whom continued to experience pain after being operated upon. Many people have reported immediate, lasting improvement from this one lesson.

PART ONE   *Sitting*

1   Sit in a chair as you normally do, comfortably. A wooden chair (or stool) or other firm chair is preferable to a more cushioned one. Don't try to "sit up straight" or exactly like the drawings, or in any other way you've been told is "right."

31

Move your head up and down, gently, as you do when saying "yes." Do that a number of times.

Sense how you make this familiar movement. Notice what happens in your chest, shoulders, upper back. If you are leaning against the back of your chair, sense any change in the contact or pressure of your back against the chair. Remember, to sense clearly, do the movement slowly and easily, and breathe freely.

Notice how far you move in each direction, the range. More important, sense the quality of movement, the ease and fluidity.

2 As you nod your head "yes," observe what you are doing spontaneously with your eyes. Are you looking forward continuously as if watching something, moving your eyes passively with your head, or actively looking downward and upward?

Continue to nod your head "yes." Look down as you lower your head and look up as you raise your head, intentionally. You can do that with your eyes closed, since there is nothing you need to see, or you can have your eyes open.

Does coordinating your head and eyes change the way you nod your head?

Pause for a moment.

3 Notice how you have been sitting. Are you leaning against the back of the chair? Are your legs crossed or asymmetrical in some way? Do both feet contact the floor, or only one?

Slide your pelvis forward a few inches so that you sit without leaning against the back of your chair. Place both feet fully on the floor.

Are you comfortable sitting without any back support, or does this seem awkward? Do what you can to sit easily, without excess effort. Remember, you can rest any time you sense strain or fatigue.

4 Nod "yes," again. Look down as you lower your head and up as you raise your head. Repeat that a number of times.

Does sitting forward with both feet on the floor affect how you nod your head? Does your head move farther or easier? Are you

Part One
Step Three

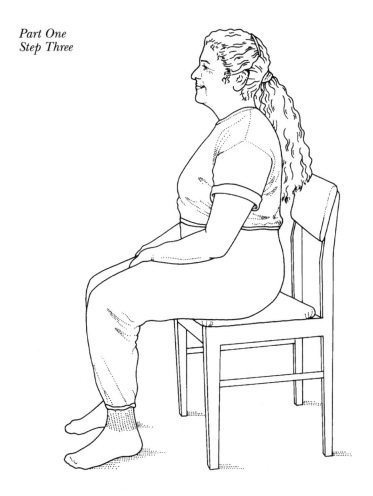

more aware of your shoulders, chest, and back? Can you sense movement further down your spine, in your mid-back or lower back? Is your pelvis moving as you nod "yes?" Is your weight shifting slightly backward or forward?

Pause. Continue to sit without leaning against the back of the chair.

5 The pelvis is a fairly complex structure. On each side is a sitting bone that somehow contacts the chair and a hip joint where the

Part One
Step Four

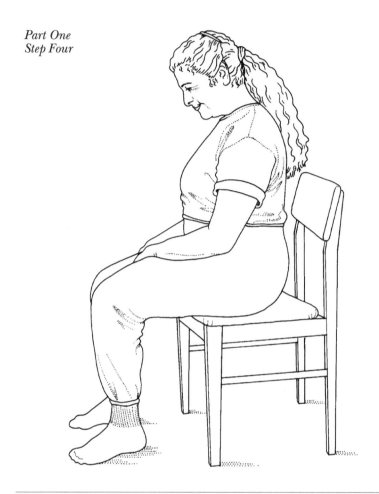

leg and pelvis meet. Most people have only a relatively vague sense of the shape of these bones and joints.

Tilt your pelvis to rock backward on your sitting bones. Then straighten your pelvis to sit up again. Do that a number of times.

You gently slump or slouch in your chair as you rock your pelvis backward. Then you straighten and become taller as you tilt your pelvis forward.

Sense how tilting your pelvis involves your hip joints and your whole spine. As your pelvis rocks backward, your back rounds

Part One
Step Five

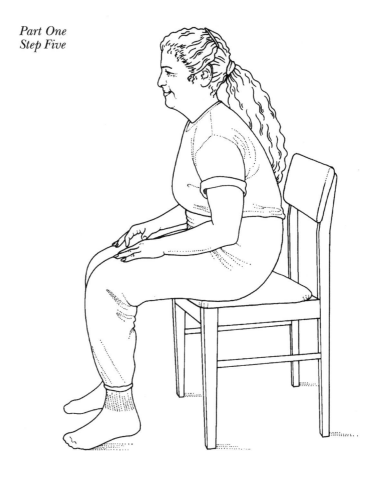

slightly toward the back of your chair. Initiate the movement from your pelvis, simply, and otherwise move more or less passively. Let your head move freely.

Notice how your sitting bones tilt or pivot. If you are on a firm chair, you may be able to sense the shape of these bones. Sense the movement in your hip joints, how your pelvis tilts relative to your legs. The largest and strongest muscles you have are those which connect your legs and pelvis.

Rest. Lean against the back of the chair if you like.

Part One
Step Six

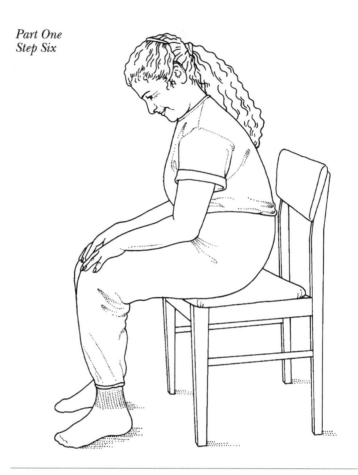

6 Sit forward, away from the back of your chair, with your feet fully on the floor.

Again, begin to nod your head "yes." Do that many times as you gently, gradually, make the movement larger. A good way to make this movement gradually larger is to think of adding one vertebra each time you nod "yes." You have seven vertebrae in your neck, twelve in your upper back and mid-back, five in your lower back, plus the sacrum and tailbones in your pelvis. Let each movement be slightly larger than the one before, as long as you are comfortable. Sense how this also enlarges the motion in your chest, upper back, and further down your spine.

Say "yes" with your whole spine. Sense the movement from the top of your head to the tip of your tail, and everywhere in between. Be sure you breathe freely as you move.

Observe how your head bends forward and your spine rounds backward as your pelvis tilts. See if you can do this so your spine makes a smooth, continuous curve from your sitting bones and tailbone, through your lower back, your mid-back and upper back, your neck, and into your head. Sense the movement in your ribs all around, in your chest, sides, and back. If you were watching yourself from the side, you would see your spine curve like the letter C, and then straighten.

Notice how you breathe as you do this movement. At what point in the movement do you breathe in, and at what point do you breathe out? Are you coordinating your breathing with the movement?

Pause briefly.

7 Say "yes" with your whole spine and deliberately coordinate this with your breathing. Breathe in as you move in one direction. Breathe out as you move in the opposite direction. A complete breath, in and out, corresponds to a complete movement, bending and straightening.

Do that 5 or 10 times, comfortably, as slowly or as quickly as you like. Notice how you are coordinating bending with breathing. In which direction are you moving when you breathe in? As you bend, are you breathing in or out?

8 Reverse the way you coordinate these movements. If you were breathing in while straightening, now breathe in while you bend and breathe out while you straighten. Do 5 or 10 movements while breathing this way.

Is this breathing pattern easier or more difficult? Are your movements smaller or larger? Sense the difference in your ribs all around, your chest and back, your abdomen, diaphragm, pelvis, and hip joints. In each of these areas, notice how changing the way you breathe affects how you move.

Pause for an instant and again reverse the way you breathe as you bend and straighten. This is how you first coordinated these movements. Did you spontaneously do it in the easier way? Or does this pattern now seem more difficult?

Let your breathing regulate the size and timing of bending and straightening. If you are breathing deeply, the movement is large or slow. The movement is smaller or faster if your breathing is not as deep. You move in one direction as long as you are breathing in, then you reverse the direction of the movement as you begin to breathe out.

Do the movement this way a few times, then reverse the coordination again. Continue to say "yes" with your entire spine, and reverse the coordination after every 2 or 3 movements.

Note that I am not telling you which way of bending and breathing is "correct." Instead, by asking you to sense several variations, I am creating conditions for you to discover which you prefer. Real learning involves experiencing, not just following directions. In this way, you are learning simultaneously to do these movements more skillfully and to be more aware and autonomous.

9 Identify which breathing pattern is easier for you right now. Continue bending and breathing in the way you prefer. Exhale completely, slowly and easily, as you move in one direction; inhale as you smoothly move in the opposite direction.

Sense how this movement involves your hip joints, pelvis, lower back, mid-back, upper back, ribs, chest, shoulders, neck, and head.

Gradually make the movement smaller. The movement may become faster as it becomes smaller, with your breathing simpler and not so deep. Do 15 or 20 movements, each smaller than the last, until the movement is so small that someone watching you would not see you moving. Continue to make this minimal movement as you breathe easily.

Notice how you are sitting now. Sense your pelvis and sitting bones, and how your head and spine relate to your pelvis. Compare this with how you were sitting at the beginning of this lesson.

PART TWO   *Lying on Your Back*

1 Lie on your back on the floor with your arms at your sides. If you use a mat, pad, or rug, it should not be uneven or overly soft. Rest.

Be aware of how you are at this moment, especially how you contact the floor. Without altering your position, sense where and how you contact the floor. Are there places where that contact seems unclear or incomplete? The more you sense now, the more you will be able to notice any changes later.

Notice how your head contacts the floor and sense the space between your neck and the floor. A small percentage of people have a very large gap there and are uncomfortable lying without a pillow. If that includes you, find a firm pillow or even a paperback book or two to place under your head so that you are comfortable.

Also, there is some space between the lower back and the floor with most people. Do you sense that? If so, notice where that gap begins and ends, and how high it might be. Take a moment to sense that as clearly as you can. Now gently slide one hand under your lower back. Did you sense the size of the gap accurately, or is it larger or smaller than you at first perceived? Is that space large enough for your forearm, your hand, your fingers only?

2 Bend your legs and place the soles of your feet flat on the floor. Your knees will be in the air. Interlace your fingers and place your hands behind your head. Be sure your hands are under the heaviest part of your head, not under your neck. Sense the weight of your head in your hands.

Lift your head, easily, two or three inches at most, and lower it. See if you can carry your head with your arms and shoulders, so that your neck remains relaxed. That is especially important if you ever experience pain or stiffness in your neck. Each time you lower your head, rest completely for an instant and sense the weight of your head and hands on the floor.

Keep this movement small and easy. I emphasize this because the movement resembles sit-ups and many people habitually strain while doing sit-ups. Here we are interested in learning, not in strengthening abdominal muscles. If you learn to be more aware

Part Two
Step Two

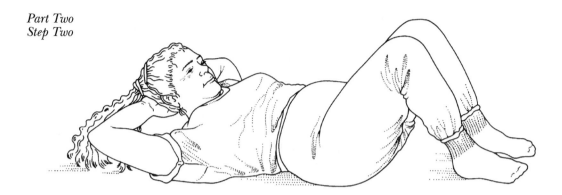

and skillful, tomorrow you will be able to do sit-ups with less effort than in the past, and with greater benefits. Remember, the less effort you use, the more you can sense and learn.

One way to make sensing and learning easier is to recall that every movement involves all of yourself. Sense your shoulders and chest, the muscles all through the abdomen and into the pelvis and hip joints as you do this movement.

3 As you continue to lift and lower your head, notice what you are doing with your arms. Are you holding them stiffly?

Move your elbows toward each other while you lift your head. Move your elbows away from each other while you lower your head.

Does moving your arms this way help you lift and lower your head more easily? Most people find that it does, but, again, I want you to see what is best for you. Experiment and see if you prefer to move your arms as you lift and lower your head or if you would rather keep your arms in the same relative position.

Rest. Lower your arms to your sides. Leave your legs bent or extend them, as you prefer. Simply lie still and do nothing.

4 Again, bend your legs so your feet are flat on the floor, interlace your fingers, and place your hands behind your head.

Lift and lower your head easily, a number of times. Use your arms and sense how all the muscles in front participate.

Part Two
Step Three

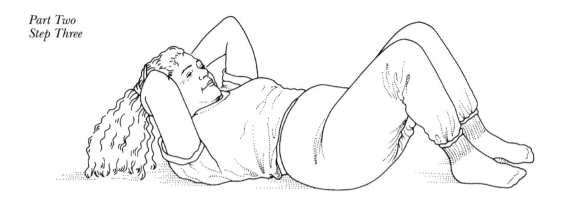

As you lift and lower your head, notice your breathing. Are you breathing in a way that somehow coordinates with the movement?

Deliberately breathe with the movement. Breathe in while you move in one direction, and breathe out while you move in the opposite direction. One complete movement, lifting and lowering your head, corresponds to one complete breath, in and out.

Pause briefly.

5 Resume the movement while breathing the opposite way. If you were breathing out while lifting your head, now breathe in while you lift and breathe out while you lower.

How does this affect the range and quality of the movement? Is this easier or more difficult?

Do a few movements breathing one way, pause, and do a few movements breathing the opposite way. Continue to lift and lower your head, pausing every 3 or 4 movements and reversing the way you breathe.

Reduce the effort as much as possible so you can more clearly sense the differences between these variations. Remember, what you do habitually always feels normal and easier at first. Be sure you rest on the floor for an instant between repetitions. With each variation, sense the range and quality of movement, the amount of effort throughout your trunk, down into your pelvis and hip joints.

Here are several other variations you may want to explore: You can breathe out as you lift and lower, and breathe in as you rest. Or the reverse, breathing in as you move and breathing out as you rest. Another possibility is to hold your breath as you move, and breathe in and out as you rest. How many sit-ups have you done in your life without being aware of your breathing or exploring ways to move more effectively?

6 Rest. Bring your arms to your sides. Extend your legs. Just be still for a few moments.

Notice how you feel now, after doing this movement. Observe how your back makes contact with the floor. Do you sense any difference from when you began this part of the lesson?

PART THREE *Lying on Your Front*

1 Roll over to lie on your front. Position your arms on the floor so that one hand is on top of the other, and rest your forehead on the upper hand. Your hands create a platform for your forehead.

Find a way to be comfortable in this position. Adjust the position of your arms, hands, and head, if you like. Some people prefer to have a pad or small pillow under the chest, belly, or pelvis.

2 Look up toward the ceiling and lift your head off your hands. Then look down toward your chin and lower your forehead onto your hands. Your eyes lead the movement of lifting and lowering your head.

As always, do this within the range that is completely comfortable. For many people, arching backward is quite unfamiliar, so keep this movement small and easy.

In this position, muscles in your back contract to lift your head, then the same muscles lengthen as your head returns to the floor. Sense, as clearly as you can, where muscles are working, in your neck, between your shoulder blades, in your mid-back, your lower back, all the way down to your pelvis and legs.

Also, notice if you are pressing your arms and hands into the floor. If you are aware and that helps, do it, but do not lift any higher than is really comfortable.

Part Three
Step One

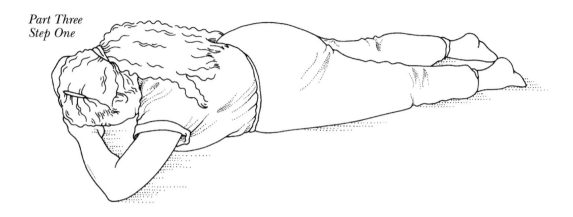

Part Three
Step Two

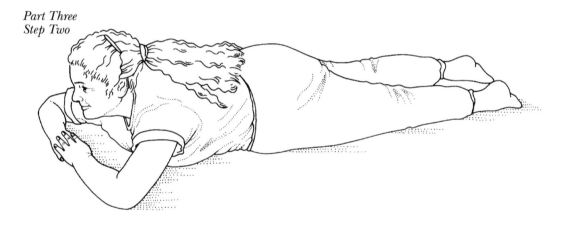

3 Continue looking up and lifting your head, then looking down and lowering your head. Rest your head on your hands for a moment each time you lower, to allow the muscles in your back to relax. Sense that.

Once again, note how you are breathing spontaneously. Do the movement a few more times to sense that.

Now deliberately coordinate lifting and lowering your head with your breathing. Breathe in as you move in one direction; breathe out as you move in the opposite direction. Do several movements breathing out as you lift your head, breathing in as you lower your head. Then pause and reverse the pattern. Breathe in as you lift your head and out as you lower.

Continue to do 2 or 3 movements breathing one way, then 2 or 3 movements breathing the opposite way. Let each movement be smooth and comfortable, in accordance with how you breathe easily. Remember to rest your head on your hands for a moment whenever you lower.

Sense the difference between these two ways of coordinating the movement with your breathing. Observe the range and quality of the movement. Which feels easier and more comfortable— breathing out as you lift and in as you lower, or breathing in as you lift and out as you lower?

Rest. Turn your head to either side and place your hands wherever you like. For a few moments, simply breathe easily and lie quietly.

4   Place one hand on top of the other again and rest your forehead on the back of the uppermost hand. Look up toward the ceiling and lift your head to follow your eyes, easily. Look down toward the floor below your chest as you lower your head. Do that a few more times, clearly sensing how your eyes direct the movement. Coordinate your breathing with the movement.

Pause.

Find a way to move your head and eyes in opposite directions. Lift your head while moving your eyes down to look at the floor; then look up toward the ceiling as you lower your head.

This movement will probably seem awkward, and your head may not lift as far. Fine. Intentionally keep the movement small. Let the movement be somewhat unsteady or poorly coordinated. As long as you are comfortable, you are learning. If you sense any holding or forcing of your breathing, pause again for a moment.

See if you can make this movement lighter and easier.

Close your eyes as you lift and lower your head while moving your eyes in the opposite direction. See if that helps you coordinate your head and eyes more easily. Do another 5 or 10 or more movements.

To do this well, your eyes and head should move continuously, reach the farthest point at the same instant, and reverse direction smoothly. If you want to learn to do this well, begin by playing and doing it poorly.

Pause.

Again, look up toward the ceiling and follow your eyes with your head. Then look down to the floor beneath your chest as you lower your head. Notice if doing the opposite movement with your eyes has helped you do this more freely and easily.

Rest. Again, position your arms wherever you like and turn your head toward either side. If you like, rest with your head turned to the opposite side from the last rest. Notice if turning your head the opposite way is more or less comfortable, or if there seems to be no difference.

5 Now place your hands on the floor near your shoulders, as if you were going to do a push-up, and face the floor. Begin to lift and lower your head again. Do not do actual push-ups, but only use your arms to assist in lifting your head. Your forearms and elbows can remain on the floor or lift slightly.

Look up toward the ceiling as you lift your head, and look toward the floor beneath your belly as you lower your head. Let your eyes move to lead your head in lifting and lowering. You can do this with your eyes open or closed.

Stay within the range that is comfortable. As before, the goal is to learn something about how to move more easily.

Sense how all of the muscles in your back work together as you lift your head, and how they lengthen as you lower your head to the floor.

Experiment with breathing in different ways as you do this larger backward movement. A few times, breathe out as you lift and in as you lower, then breathe in as you lift and out as you lower.

Sense how each way of breathing assists or inhibits movement. Do each variation a few more times and note any differences as clearly as you can. As you do this backward bending, which way of breathing is easier?

Part Three
Step Five

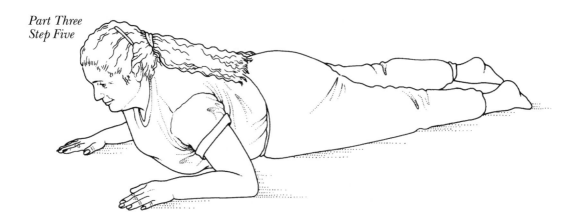

6 Gradually make the movement larger, while continuing to breathe in the way you sense to be easier. Use your arms, shoulders, and all the muscles in your back, from your head and neck through to your pelvis and hip joints. Make the movement as large as comfortable.

Most of us spend a great deal of time sitting in cars, leaning over desks or tables, and in other positions that round the spine forward. These backward movements provide a valuable—sometimes necessary—counterbalance. If you have any pain or problem with your back, be especially attentive while you do this; lift only as high as comfortable and easy.

7 Roll onto your back and rest. Lie still for a moment. Be aware of how you feel. Sense how you contact the floor. Is anything different from before? Do you have a more complete awareness of your back and how you contact the floor?

You may sense more space beneath your lower back than before. If so, simply be aware. A larger space simply indicates that the backward movement has left some residual contraction in those muscles. The next part of the lesson will relieve that. Right now, simply be aware of how large a space there is between your lower back and the floor.

What have you learned so far about breathing and bending? When you were sitting, did you find it easier to breathe out when bending forward and in when straightening? When lying on your back, did you prefer to breathe out or in as you lifted your head? And when on your front, which was easier?

How does breathing and bending backward relate to breathing and bending forward? Is there some logical pattern, some reason you can find as to what is easier and why? Think about this, but do not be too attached to any particular answer. As you become more aware, the pattern will be clear and you may discover that what seems easier now is only habitual. You interfere with learning whenever you insist too soon on one answer.

Remember, resting is important for learning. Take time to learn.

PART FOUR *Lying on Your Back*

1   Bend your legs so your feet are flat on the floor. Lift your right foot off the floor, and take hold of your right leg below the knee with your right hand. Hold the leg below the knee on the outside, not behind the knee. Hold your left leg with your left hand in the same way. Keep your arms straight and let your lower legs hang downward easily.

2   Bend your arms and bring your knees toward your chest. Then straighten your arms and move your legs away.

Sense the movement in your hip joints and pelvis. Notice what you are doing with your abdomen and all the muscles in front. As always, make the movement smoothly and gently and eliminate any excess effort.

Sense the movement in your arms, shoulders, hip joints, pelvis, abdomen, and all the muscles in your front. Are you breathing easily? Did you spontaneously coordinate your breathing with the movement? If so, how?

3   Deliberately coordinate the movement of your legs with your breathing. Do a few movements breathing out as you fold your knees toward your chest and breathing in as you move your knees away. Then do a few movements breathing the opposite way. Continue to move your knees toward your chest and away, reversing your breathing after every 2 or 3 movements. Leave your head on the floor as you do this.

*Part Four
Step One*

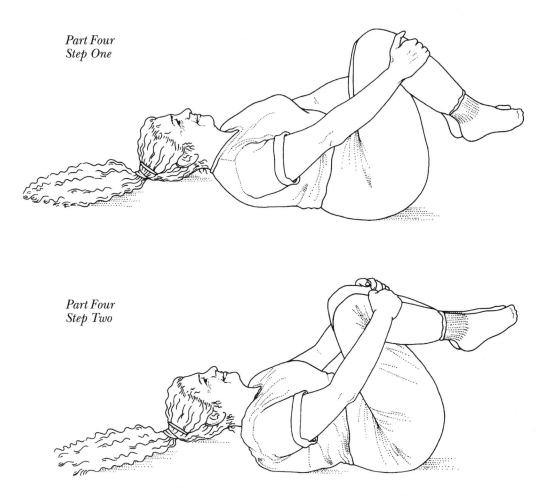

*Part Four
Step Two*

Again, notice how these variations affect the range and quality of the movement. Discover all you can about which variation is easier, and how.

While breathing in the way that seems easier, bring your knees toward your chest and away a few more times.

If you want to—and if it is easy and you remember to make the movement with minimal effort—lift your head as your knees come toward your face and lower your head as your knees go away. Your head and knees move toward each other and apart. If lifting your head is at all difficult, simply imagine lifting your head.

Each time you bring your knees toward your chest, muscles all through your front, from your shoulders to your hip joints, contract. Sense what happens in your back at the same time. Can you detect any lengthening there? Does the pressure of your back against the floor change as you move? If you are breathing easily and moving comfortably, you may sense that.

Release your knees, extend your legs, rest.

Has your contact with the floor changed?

4 Bend your legs so your feet are flat on the floor again. Notice how your legs stand and where your feet are relative to your pelvis. Slide your feet a bit farther from or nearer to one another and see if they stand more easily. Slide your feet a bit farther from, then nearer to, your pelvis. Can you position your feet and knees so that they stand effortlessly?

Interlace your fingers and place your hands behind your head. Be sure your hands are under the heaviest part of your head, not just your neck.

Recall when you lifted your head with your hands in this position before. Now think through all you have discovered about how to do this movement in the easiest possible way. How do you want to breathe? What can you do with your arms? Where might you be looking as you move?

When you are ready, lift and lower your head. Make this movement as smooth and easy as you can. Sense how muscles in your arms, shoulders, chest, abdomen, pelvis, and hip joints contract together. At the same time, sense any lengthening in your back muscles or other changes in the way your back presses the floor.

To check that you are doing this in the easiest way, try some variations and see if they make the movement more difficult. Lift and lower your head a few times while deliberately keeping your elbows fixed and apart. Intentionally breathe opposite to the way you are now breathing. Do these changes inhibit or interfere with how you move?

Part Four
Step Four

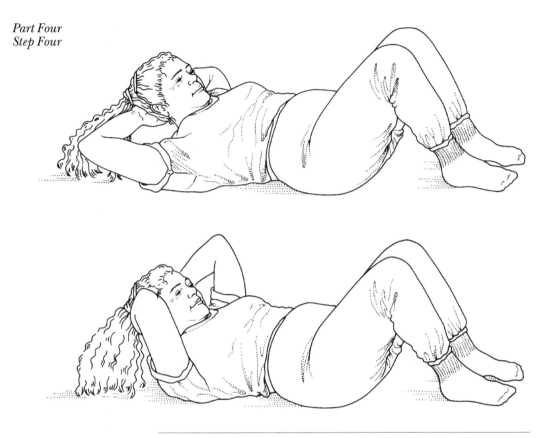

Lift and lower your head a few more times in the way that seems easiest.

Sense the range and quality of movement everywhere.

5   Continue to lift your head with your arms, easily, and notice where you are looking as you do that. How do you move your eyes? What do you see?

As you lift your head each time, look toward your pelvis and chest. Look up toward the ceiling as you lower your head. See if you can move your eyes smoothly. You can do that with your eyes open or closed. Coordinate the movement of your eyes with the lifting and lowering of your head.

Pause.

Now move your eyes in the opposite direction. Look upward, toward the ceiling, as you lift your head. Look toward your pelvis and chest as you lower your head. Make this movement as smoothly coordinated as you can. Remember to breathe easily, harmoniously.

Pause again.

Again, lift and lower your head with your arms while looking in the direction in which you are moving. Sense the coordination between your head and your eyes. Notice the range and quality of this movement now. Has varying the movement of your eyes somehow helped you move your head more easily?

Rest briefly, with your legs remaining bent.

6 Again, use your arms and everything you have learned to lift and lower your head. Each time you do this, if it is easy, simultaneously lift your feet off the floor and move your knees toward your elbows. As your knees move toward your elbows, also move your elbows toward your knees. Then, as you lower your head, move your knees and elbows apart and return your feet to the floor.

Be sure you do this comfortably, with no excess effort. Breathe with the movement, as you have been learning, harmoniously.

And rest for an instant each time your head and feet are on the floor.

Sense how all of the muscles in front work as you fold yourself. Notice how muscles are engaging in your arms and shoulders, your upper chest and ribs, your abdomen and pelvis and hip joints. As all of those muscles contract, sense how, simultaneously, muscles all along your back lengthen. Be aware of the reverse as you lower your head and elbows to the floor and move your knees away.

7 Rest. Extend your legs or leave them bent, with your arms at your sides. For a few moments, do nothing. Simply breathe easily and sense how you contact the floor now.

8 Interlace your fingers in front of your face, where you can see them. Notice how one thumb is on top of the other or closer to your face, then, starting with one forefinger, all of the fingers

51

Part Four
Step Six

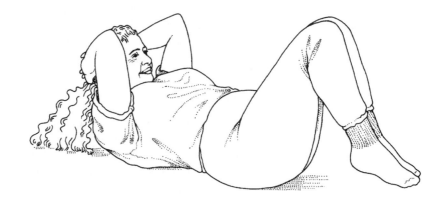

alternate, left, right, left, right, and so on. Unlace your fingers and interlace them in the opposite position. If the left thumb and forefinger were above their counterparts on the right, now place the right ones on top.

Your hands will look the same, superficially, but if you have never done this before it will feel quite different. Some people find this extremely strange, as if their hands are someone else's. You may want to simply look at your hands for a moment while they are interlaced in this unfamiliar way. If you like, switch from one to the other a few times.

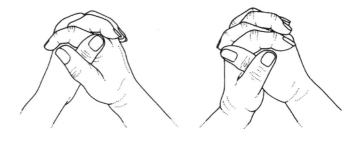

9 With your fingers interlaced in this nonhabitual way, place your hands behind your head.

Use your arms, shoulders, and all the muscles in your front to lift and lower your head. Breathe easily. Look in the direction in which you are moving.

This small change in the way you interlace your fingers may alter your experience of this very familiar movement. When you change one element in this way, with awareness, a fundamental reorganizing occurs throughout the sensory and motor areas of the brain.

As you continue to lift and lower your head, consider what you have learned about yourself and how to do this simple, easy movement. With this or any movement, small changes in how you breathe, move your eyes, even how you interlace your fingers, can affect both range and quality. When you are aware, you can move comfortably and effectively and do whatever you want.

Pause momentarily. Change your fingers back to your habitual way of interlacing them. Continue to lift and lower your head.

Notice how easily you lift and lower your head when aware and moving harmoniously. Compare how you do this now with how you moved at the start of this lesson. Is this easier than before? Do you make a larger movement with less effort? Do you feel more comfortable and coordinated?

10 Rest. Extend your legs and bring your arms to your sides. Sense your head, neck, shoulders, upper back, mid-back, lower back, legs, and arms.

Notice how you contact the floor now, in the area around your lower back and generally. Is there any gap between your lower back and the floor? If so, is that space smaller or larger than before? Do you sense your contact with the floor more clearly and completely? Does the floor seem softer and more accommodating?

Also notice your breathing. Sense the range and quality of movement in your ribs in your front and sides and back, with both inhaling and exhaling. Are you breathing differently from usual, more slowly, completely, and easily, perhaps?

Rest for a few more minutes. Remember, the learning occurs through this process of distinguishing differences. Be aware of any changes in how you are now compared with how you were when you began this lesson or other times.

PART FIVE *Concluding*

1 Think about what would be the easiest way to stand. How could you roll onto either side and then stand with the least effort? See if you can discover a way to stand with the same awareness and comfort you experienced while doing the movements on the floor. This is an important aspect of the lesson. If you just stand quickly, you may re-create habitual ways of moving.

When you are ready, slowly, smoothly, comfortably, roll onto either side and stand.

Sense how you stand now. Compare how you are standing now with the way you normally stand. Do you feel taller, lighter, straighter? Do you stand with less effort? Perhaps you feel shorter and heavier? Simply compare, without judging what is good or desirable.

2 Walk. Notice the movement in your pelvis and hip joints. Sense the mobility throughout your trunk as you walk and breathe easily. Do you notice any change in how you walk now compared with your habitual way of walking? Remember, the more you can be aware, the more you will learn. It may take a few moments for you to sense differences, but even a relatively subtle change can have a profound effect over time.

3 Again, sit without leaning against the back of your chair, with your feet fully on the floor.

Breathe out and bend, rounding your spine backward toward the chair as your head and pelvis move forward and toward each other. Breathe in and straighten, returning fluidly to a neutral, vertical position.

Make this movement as large and free as comfortable. As you bend, look downward, toward your chest and chin. As you straighten, see if you can move your eyes smoothly, to look at the wall in front of you. Coordinate your eyes, your bending, and your breathing.

Sense the movement in your pelvis and hip joints, your abdomen and lower back, your chest and ribs all around, your mid-back, upper back, shoulders, neck, and head. Notice how all the muscles, front and back, work harmoniously.

Part Five
Step Three

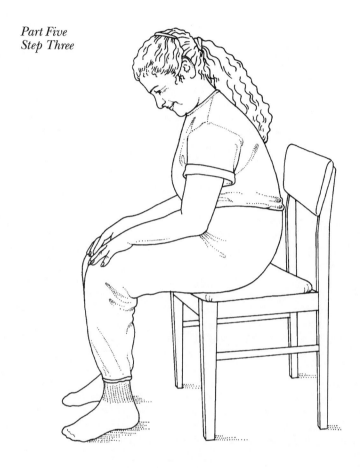

Compare the range and quality of this movement now with when you did it earlier.

I encourage you to explore and refine these bending and breathing movements in many ways. While it is easier to learn when sitting on a firm seat without back support and with your feet flat on the floor, you can explore these movements anywhere, adjusting the movement in accordance with your seat and situation. You may want to do bending and breathing movements while sitting in the car, eating, or at the movies, perhaps making the movements so small that people around do not notice. You might also play with these movements while sitting on the floor

55

Maria was referred to me following a back injury, which had not improved in spite of several months each of chiropractic treatment and physical therapy. The orthopedic surgeon who sent her to me said he could not find anything objectively wrong; he suspected she was just not motivated to improve and might be exaggerating her complaints while hoping for an insurance settlement. Although I did not quarrel with him at the time, I generally question such judgments. I believe people become or appear to be unmotivated only when they are unaware and do not know how to act comfortably and effectively.

It was a beautiful June day at three o'clock in the afternoon when Maria first walked into my office. Maria, 23 years old, slender and pretty, had been working as a hotel maid when she slipped in a bathroom and hurt herself. From the way she walked and sat, I could see immediately that muscles throughout her trunk were tight and her breathing was quite shallow. She seemed to lack any sense of how her head and pelvis connect or of how breathing involves moving. I asked what she would be doing that afternoon if the doctor had not sent her to see me, and Maria told me she would be home watching television.

I taught Maria the preceding lesson during that first visit, guiding her through the movements by touch as well as with verbal directions. As we finished, I asked Maria to practice at home, and she agreed to do so. Then I told her, "I want you to do this while you watch television. When the program is on you can make a small movement, gently tilting your pelvis to sense some easy bending as you breathe. When the commercials come on, Maria, make the movement as large as possible. Breathe fully and curve your spine as comfortably and completely as you can. Look up at the ceiling and down toward yourself as you do that."

Within two weeks, after only a few more lessons, Maria was almost completely free of pain. A few months later, I saw her at a supermarket downtown and she told me that she had returned to college and was planning to complete her associate's degree.

in various positions, or leaning back on a sofa, with your legs crossed or resting on something.

Remember, healing comes with increasing awareness, not from doing movements of any particular size or rate or number of repetitions, nor from simply stretching or strengthening muscles. Any time you sense strain or stiffness in your back or your neck or anywhere, you can benefit from bending and breathing and being more aware.

Lesson Two

Turning and Twisting

People often come to me complaining of pain or difficulty turning their heads. While some describe a whiplash or other injury, many tell me, "I don't know what caused it. I just woke up this way one morning, stiff and unable to turn." Then, to demonstrate how limited the movement in the neck is, many people deliberately hold the back and shoulders absolutely straight while turning the head from side to side.

I generally respond by imitating the way the person is moving and explain that no one can turn the head freely while stiffening the shoulders and holding the breath. Somehow, most people seem to believe the head and neck should move independently of the shoulders, chest, and back.

In this lesson, you will learn how turning your head involves your shoulders, pelvis, eyes, and all of yourself.

Part One *Sitting*

1 Sit in a chair as you normally do, comfortably. Turn your head left and right, simply.

As you turn, notice what you do. You can feel the turning in your neck, of course. Also sense your shoulders, your chest, your upper back. Where are you moving? Where are you not moving?

Notice how far you turn your head without any effort. Choose some point on the wall to indicate the extent of your turning in each direction. Remember that point, and at the end of the lesson you can use it as a reference to see if you turn further.

2 A few more times, turn your head left and right. Sense what you do with your eyes as you turn your head.

Are your eyes moving so that you actually look from one side to the other? Or are your eyes immobile relative to your head, as when staring at your nose? Perhaps you kept your eyes focused on something in front of you, so that your head moved relative to your eyes. Simply be aware of whatever you did without thinking.

PART TWO   *Lying on the Floor*

1 Lie on the floor and rest, with your arms at your sides and your legs extended.

Sense how you are right now. Notice where you make contact with the floor and where you feel any spaces or gaps. Recall how you sensed the floor when you completed the previous lesson, and notice any differences between then and now. Along with sensing your contact with the floor, notice the quality of your awareness and how clearly you sense yourself. Take a few moments to sense how you are now. Remember, learning occurs by perceiving differences. The more clearly you sense how you are now, the more differences you will discover later.

If the space behind your neck is large and your head hangs uncomfortably, place a firm pillow or paperback book under your head. Be sure that anything you use is firm enough to provide a reliable surface; a soft pillow will interfere with your ability to sense clearly how you are moving. If you are comfortable with no pillow, that is best.

2 Turn your head left and right. If you do that simply, the back of your head rolls on the floor and your chin moves toward one shoulder and then toward the other shoulder. If the back of your head slides on the floor you are doing more work than when simply rolling. Continue turning your head, making the movement smoother, simpler, easier.

Part Two
Step Three

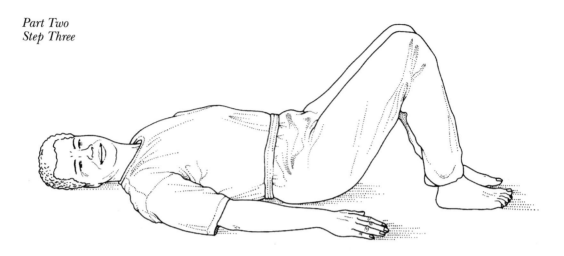

Sense your head, your neck, your chest, your upper back. Notice how far and how freely your head turns without any effort.

Pause.

3 Bend your legs so that your feet are flat on the floor, with your knees in the air. Resume turning your head, the back of your head rolling on the floor.

Does having the legs bent alter the movement in your neck? Some people find that they turn their heads more easily. Bending your legs tilts your pelvis slightly, altering the position and activity in the muscles there and along your spine. Can you detect whether a change at one end of the spine affects the movement at the opposite end?

That is fairly subtle, and most people will not notice any difference at first. You will be more aware of those connections after completing this lesson.

As you turn your head, sense the changing contact between your head and the floor, that rolling motion. Notice the turning in your neck and any movement in your shoulders. How far down your spine can you detect the rolling of your head?

Rest for a moment. Sense your head, neck, shoulders, and how you contact the floor.

4 Extend your arms toward the ceiling. Place your palms together so that your arms form a triangle with your chest.

Move your arms left and right, keeping your back in continuous partial contact with the floor, neither sliding nor lifting. Keep your hands together and your elbows and wrists more or less straight. I say more or less straight so you do not stiffen. If you slide your hands, bend your wrists, or bend your elbows, the movement in your shoulders will not be as clear. Also, see if you can keep your arms perpendicular to your torso, not angling down toward your knees or up toward your nose.

As you move your arms from side to side, notice where this movement occurs in your shoulders, chest, back, and neck. Most of us have only a vague notion of how the shoulder is structured and moves. The head of the upper arm bone is a ball shape that fits into a socket that is part of the shoulder blade. Sense how moving your arms from side to side involves moving your shoulder blade, how one shoulder blade lifts while the opposite shoulder blade presses the floor.

Your collarbones, or clavicles, also move with your arms, because the collarbone attaches to the shoulder blade. At the other end of the collarbone is an attachment to the breastbone, the sternum. That joint, where the collarbone meets the sternum, is actually quite mobile, or can be. Even after studying anatomy, people rarely sense or appreciate how moving the arm involves mobility there. Anyone who has difficulty with arm movements, including tennis elbow and carpal tunnel syndrome, has restricted the mobility in the shoulder blades and collarbones.

Continue to move your arms from side to side and sense the movement in your shoulder blades, collarbones, and sternum. Notice how your ribs participate, in your chest, sides, and back. Be aware of places that move easily, and places that seem stiff or restricted. As you become more aware, stiffness will often disappear spontaneously.

Remember to breathe easily. Any holding or forcing of the breath will interfere with the mobility of the ribs, sternum, collarbones, and shoulder blades. When you move these central

Part Two
Step Four

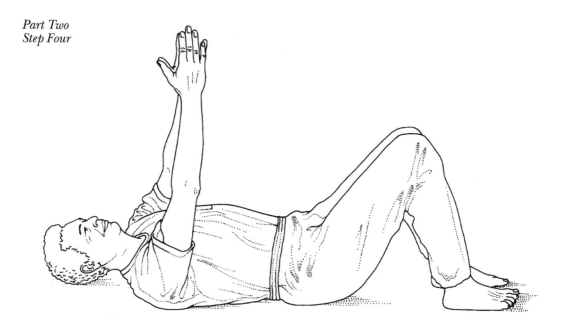

areas more freely, you improve the strength and mobility of your arms, elbows, wrists, hands, and fingers.

Pause. Lower your arms to your sides.

5   Simply turn your head left and right again. Does your head move more easily now, after doing the movement with your arms?

There are many reasons why your head may roll more freely. The major muscles that turn your head attach at their opposite ends to the shoulder blades, collarbones, or sternum. Rolling your head uses these muscles in one way, while tilting your arms as you were just doing uses the same muscles from the opposite end. Improving any movement brings many benefits.

Rest briefly. Lie quietly and breathe easily. Sense how you contact the floor.

6   Bend your legs so your feet are flat on the floor. Leave your arms at your sides.

Part Two
Step Six

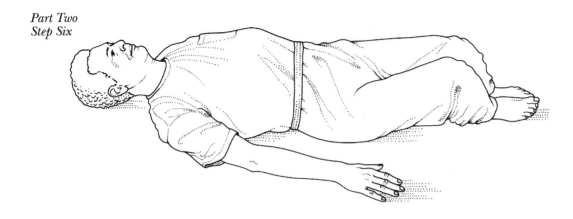

Tilt your knees to the left and to the right, simply. Do that so your feet remain in continuous partial contact with the floor, neither sliding nor lifting. Your feet move like hinges on the floor, the inside of one foot and the outside of the other foot leave the floor as your legs tilt to either side. Your legs remain more or less parallel to each other.

These specific constraints help you be more aware of how you move your hip joints and pelvis. Random movements may be fun and feel good, and they are certainly preferable to immobility, but they generally fail to facilitate learning. I carefully described the position of your arms in the previous movement for the same reason, to provide specific constraints to help you become more aware and learn.

As you tilt your knees, sense how your pelvis rolls, one side lifting as the other side presses into the floor. Notice how the rolling in your pelvis also rotates vertebrae in your lower back, and this motion is transmitted through your back from one vertebra to the next. Also, sense the movement in your ribs on each side. Notice when and where your ribs lift from the floor or lower again, and how they squeeze together or fan apart.

How far up your spine can you detect movement? Is anything happening in your neck and head? Do not try to make any movement there, just notice what happens spontaneously. Does your head turn, tilt, or twist?

The position of your feet also affects the movement in your hip joints and pelvis. Mobility will be impaired if your feet are too close together or too far apart, too near or too far from your pelvis. Experiment and see if you can find the position for your feet that best allows you to tilt your legs and roll your pelvis. Remember to breathe freely as you explore these differences.

7 Pause with your knees pointing toward the ceiling and your feet flat on the floor.

Turn your head left and right again, simply, just a few times. Has doing the movement with your legs and pelvis affected the mobility of your neck and head? Does your head roll more easily now?

Rest. Extend your legs and lie still. Do nothing for a moment.

Sense how you are now. Has there been any change from when you began this lesson? Notice how you contact the floor. Also, observe the mental image you have of yourself. Has that picture become more detailed?

PART THREE *Moving Your Eyes*

1 Bend your legs so your feet are flat on the floor. Begin to move only your eyes left and right. You can do this with your eyes closed or open, although you will probably sense the movement more clearly if your eyes are closed.

See if you can move your eyes more smoothly and continuously. At first, most people find the movement of the eyes somewhat jumpy or irregular. Reduce the effort and see if you can iron out any wrinkles. Be sure you breathe easily; the movement of the eyes is subtle, and concentrating in habitual ways may involve holding the breath. If the movement seems perfectly smooth, do it more slowly.

Move your eyes left and right many times, easily.

2 Imagine some object moving from left to right and back. Follow that imaginary object with your eyes. It begins off to one side, lifts smoothly, arcs over your head, and then lowers on the other side. Imagine something you enjoy looking at. It may be a butterfly, a satellite, or a star, blue, silver, or red, and you might imagine something different for the return journey. Or you might picture a rainbow, and move your eyes from one end of the rainbow to the other. Your eyes, closed or open, follow that imaginary object up one side, across the middle, and down on the other side.

Continue to follow that imaginary object with your eyes, many times. See if you can make the movement gradually smoother and simpler. Sense that your neck and shoulders are loose, and be attentive to breathing freely.

Do your eyes move more smoothly and easily when following an imaginary object? Contrast how your eyes move now with how they moved before I suggested you imagine watching some object.

3 Begin to turn your head along with your eyes. As you look to the left, turn your head to the left. As you look to the right, turn your head to the right. Your head and your eyes move smoothly together from side to side. Continue to move your eyes to follow some imaginary object, with your eyes open or closed, as you like. As always, be attentive to breathing freely as you make the movement, simply and easily.

Sense how your head moves now, coordinating with your eyes. Compare how your head moves now with before. Does your head turn more smoothly, or farther, when you intentionally move your eyes in this way?

4 Rest. Sense your head, neck, and shoulders, and how you contact the floor. Also notice any change in your general awareness and how you sense yourself.

When watching that imaginary object, how far away from yourself did you imagine it to be—ten inches, ten yards, one hundred yards? Typically, people imagine an object at whatever distance they see most clearly. If you are nearsighted or farsighted, you probably imagined that object to be near or far, accordingly. Did you?

The fine muscles that focus the eyes coordinate with the larger muscles that move the eyes. This is necessary and reasonable, since we normally move and focus the eyes simultaneously.

Furthermore, all of these muscles coordinate with the still larger muscles that move the head. When trying to see something extremely small or distant, people squint and strain many muscles, and learning to relax those muscles and move your head and eyes more effectively can help you see more clearly. I have worked with a number of people who improved their vision and were able to stop wearing glasses.

If you want to improve your vision, there are many Feldenkrais lessons that specifically address doing so. You can also do each of the lessons in this book with more awareness of how you move and focus your eyes. Lesson One, *Bending and Breathing*, involved up and down movements with your eyes and head, and you may want to review that lesson and apply what you have just been doing with your eyes closed and following an imaginary object. You can similarly explore arcs, circles, and other patterns. Even if your vision is generally good, you will almost definitely discover that you have been habitually straining in various ways that affect your eyes. As you learn to move your eyes more easily, you may be surprised at how much more clearly and easily you can see.

PART FOUR   *Integrating*

1 Once again, bend your legs so your feet are flat on the floor. Extend your arms toward the ceiling, with your palms together and your wrists and elbows more or less straight. Move your arms left and right while turning your head in the same direction.

Notice what you are doing with your eyes. Are they moving with the head and arms? Do that deliberately. Look right as you move your head and arms to the right, and look left as you move your head and arms to the left. Your eyes move with your head and your arms, left and right, all smoothly coordinating. Breathe freely.

Keep your knees more or less in the middle, pointed toward the ceiling. Your pelvis and knees may move a bit, but if you roll your pelvis, you will not be moving within your trunk.

Sense the movement throughout your trunk, in your ribs on both sides, your spine, your shoulder blades.

Part Four
Step One

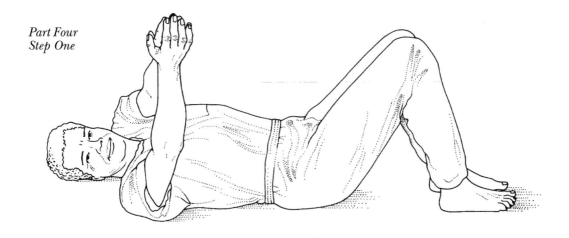

Part Four
Step Two

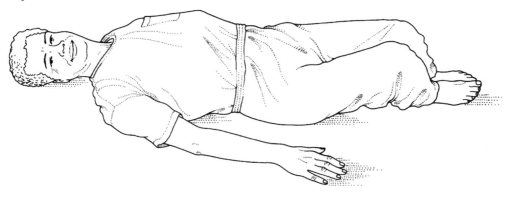

Pause and lower your arms to your sides. Leave your legs bent, your feet flat on the floor.

2 Tilt your knees left and right while turning your head and eyes in the same direction. See if you can do this as an integrated act of your head and pelvis, not as two separate movements. Both ends of your spine move together. Breathe freely.

Notice what you are doing with your shoulders. Do they remain completely still, or does one shoulder blade lift as you tilt your knees to either side? Sense the movement everywhere, in your ribs all around, in your front, sides, and back.

3 Rest. Extend your legs. Notice how you feel now. Do you contact the floor differently than before? Are you more aware of your shoulders, shoulder blades, spine, pelvis, and hip joints?

PART FIVE   *Differentiating*

1 Bend your legs so your feet are flat on the floor again. Tilt your knees to the right while you turn your head to the left, then do the reverse. Your head and legs move in opposite directions. See if you can make this a simple, integrated movement.

Be attentive to your breathing as you do this. If this seems awkward, make the movement smaller or slower and it will soon become easier. Alternatively, simply have fun doing it awkwardly, as long as you are aware, or find ways to make any awkwardness intentional.

Sense how this involves a twisting movement in your chest, sides and back, and in your ribs all around. Notice whether your arms and shoulder blades lift at all from the floor.

Be aware of your eyes. Are you moving your eyes passively as you turn your head, actively looking in the direction of your turning, keeping your eyes fixed on the ceiling, or some combination of these? Continue to move your head and knees in opposite directions and see if you can move your eyes in ways that improve the quality of this movement.

If this is nicely coordinated, your head and knees will face the ceiling at the same moment as they cross in the center of the movement. Your head and knees will also reach the end of their respective movements at the same instant.

Pause briefly and rest. Keep your legs bent.

2 Extend your arms toward the ceiling, with your palms together and your wrists and elbows more or less straight. Now move your head and your arms in opposite directions.

Part Five
Step One

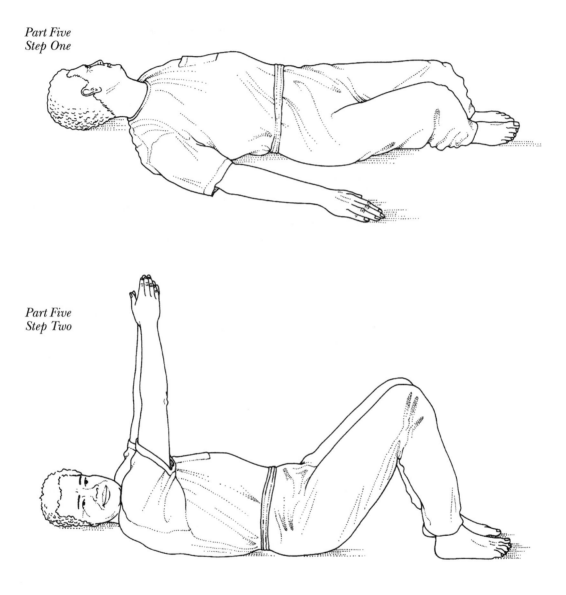

Part Five
Step Two

See if you can coordinate your head and arms so they cross in the middle and reach the furthest point in each direction at the same instant. Ideally, both your head and arms move continuously, neither slowing nor accelerating. If you want, adjust the size of the movement with your arms, your head, or both.

Sense the movement in your shoulders, shoulder blades, collarbones, and neck.

Are your eyes moving with your head, remaining fixed on the ceiling, looking at your arms? You might do any of these, with your eyes open or closed, since there is nothing you need to look at.

Rest for a moment. Bring your arms to your sides. Keep your legs bent, with your feet flat on the floor.

3 Now move your eyes and your head in opposite directions. Start slowly, breathe easily, and you will find that this is really quite simple.

To make this easier, smile. The more you enjoy this silly movement, the easier it will be and the more you will learn. Perhaps you can recall a joke you heard recently as you continue the movement.

If you find that you are straining, holding your breath, or having any difficulty, cheat. Turn your head to the right, but only 15 or 20 degrees, and leave your head there. Then look to the left as far as you can and pause for an instant. Now, at the same moment, move your head and your eyes to the center. While doing that you are moving your head and eyes simultaneously in opposite directions. Do that again, more slowly, starting from the other side, and this time continue to move your head and eyes after they reach the center. In this way, you will soon learn to move your head and eyes smoothly in opposite directions.

Like interlacing the fingers in the nonhabitual fashion, which you did in the first lesson, this is a way to disrupt habitual patterns. Coordinating the head and eyes is even more fundamental neurologically, so learning to do this movement easily can be an extremely effective way to assist in learning anything.

Move your head and eyes in opposite directions playfully, without any concern for the quality of the movement. Do it slowly or quickly, smoothly or awkwardly, many times. You might also play with following an imaginary object as you do it.

Rest. Lie still and do nothing for a few moments.

Notice how you feel after this silly movement, physically, emotionally, mentally. Sense how you contact the floor and the quality of your awareness. Was it fun? Did you learn anything?

4 Bend your legs again and extend your arms toward the ceiling with your wrists and elbows more or less straight. Now move your arms and legs in opposite directions.

Sense the movement in your ribs all around, your chest, back, and sides. Notice what happens in your shoulder blades and along your spine, from your pelvis at one end to your head at the other. How is your head moving?

See if you can coordinate your arms and legs so that they cross in the middle and reach the extreme points in their respective movements at the same moment. As always, be aware and breathe freely.

As you continue this movement, deliberately move your head and eyes in the same direction as your arms. Your eyes, head, and arms move in one direction as your legs move in the opposite direction.

Notice the range and quality of movement in your eyes, head, shoulders, and legs. Do what you can to make that simple and easy.

5 Continue to move your legs in one direction, your arms in the opposite direction, and your head with your arms. Now move your eyes with your legs. Your head and arms go one way as your eyes and legs go the opposite way. You look in the direction toward which your knees are tilting.

If this feels awkward, good. If you could do it perfectly the first time, there would be nothing for you to learn. Just make the movement as smooth and pleasant as you can. Have fun, especially if you feel uncoordinated while doing this. Be sure you are breathing easily.

See if you can do the movement with your legs, arms, and head continuously, and, after every 3 or 4 movements, switch what you are doing with your eyes. Your eyes move with your knees for a while, then your eyes move with your head and arms.

Part Five
Step Four

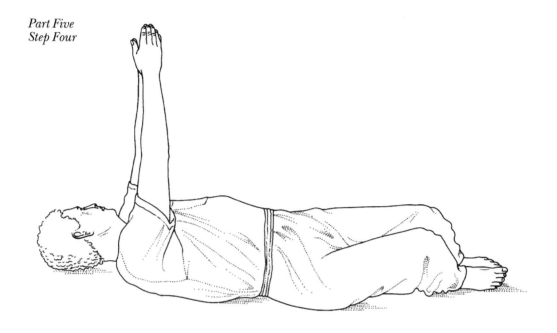

If you hold your breath as you make that shift, fine—if you are aware of doing so.

Rest briefly, with your arms at your sides. If you want to, also extend your legs.

6 Once more, bend your legs and extend your arms toward the ceiling with your wrists and elbows more or less straight.

Move your arms and legs in opposite directions, slowly, and move your head and eyes with your legs. Your legs, head, and eyes move in one direction as your arms move in the opposite direction. Do that a number of times, gradually making the movement easier and more coordinated.

Your head and pelvis turn in the same direction, rotating your spine from one end to the other. Your shoulder blades move in the opposite direction. Sense the movement in your upper back, between your shoulder blades. Remember, you will sense more when you reduce the effort. Breathe easily, to allow your ribs to move more freely in your back.

Part Five
Step Six

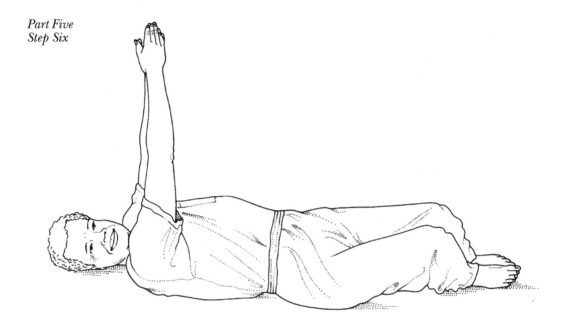

7 Continue moving your arms and legs in opposite directions, with your head turning in the same direction as your legs. Move your eyes with your arms. Your eyes and arms move one way, while your head and legs move the opposite way.

Learning always involves some confusion as we let go of the known and habitual to try something unfamiliar. Do this movement badly—as long as you are comfortable. If you allow yourself to do it badly at first, you will soon find yourself becoming better.

8 After your arms and legs move to each side 2 or 3 times, reverse the movement of your eyes, or your head, or both. Continue doing that, changing the pattern after every few movements.

Play with doing this more smoothly, simply, easily, in many variations. See if you can reverse your eyes or head without disturbing the movement of your legs and arms. Remember to smile and breathe easily.

9 Rest. Lie still. Extend your legs. Do you yawn or sigh? If so, it shows that you were not breathing as freely as you might have while doing these movements. Breathe easily as you rest.

How do you feel after this silly business? Are you more present, more alert, more relaxed? Are you lying more comfortably on the floor? Notice any change from before, both in how you contact the floor and in your awareness.

PART SIX *Reintegrating*

1 Bend your legs so your feet are flat on the floor. Leave your arms at your sides. Move your knees left and right.

Compare this movement now with when you first did it. Sense how this rolls your pelvis and involves your spine, your ribs on both sides, your chest, shoulders, neck, and head. Do your legs tilt more easily than before? Do they tilt farther? How does the movement of your head compare with before? Is it freer and more spontaneous? Notice any differences.

2 Pause with your knees in the middle. Extend your arms toward the ceiling with your palms together. Move your arms left and right.

How does this compare with when you did it earlier in the lesson? Do your arms go farther? Do your shoulder blades lift more easily? Do you have a clearer understanding of your ribs, chest, shoulders, shoulder blades, and collarbones?

Sense how the movement is transmitted through the spine down to your pelvis and legs, and up through your neck to your head.

3 Rest. Lower your arms. Now simply turn your head left and right. Compare this movement with when you began the lesson.

Notice how turning your head involves your shoulders, your chest, your back. Be aware of yourself everywhere while doing this—your lower back, pelvis, legs—where you are moving and where you may be mostly still.

Observe what your eyes are doing. Are you spontaneously looking where you turn? Sense how you move your eyes.

Pause, with your head in the middle.

4 Look left and right. Do that with your eyes closed and sense the range and quality of the movement. Then open your eyes and notice how much of the room you see.

Continue to look left and right, with your eyes open or closed, and sense how this movement involves your head, shoulders, pelvis, and everywhere else. When you are aware, relaxed and comfortable everywhere, your eyes move more freely than they can if you are straining or stiffening in any way. Your pelvis and shoulders may not be moving or doing anything to assist you in looking left and right, but they are always present.

5 Rest. Extend your legs. Lie still. How do you feel? Are you more comfortable than usual? Are you more aware? Is your image of yourself more detailed?

Compare how you are now with how you were when you first lay down. Do you contact the floor in more places? Do you have a better sense of yourself, a more detailed mental picture? That self-image may be more than visual. It may include kinesthetic sensations, pulsing, tingling, or other sensations in the surface of the skin or in the joints of the skeleton.

Allow enough rest time to sense whatever may be happening.

6 Now slowly roll toward one side and back. Then roll toward the other side and back. Sense what you do as you roll left or right. Continue gently rolling from one side to the other, sensing your eyes, head, shoulders, and pelvis.

Pause for a moment. Think about how you might extend that rolling to go smoothly onto your side and up to standing. After a few moments, find a way to do that. Roll to stand as smoothly and fluidly as you can.

7 Notice how you stand. Do you feel taller, straighter, lighter? Perhaps you seem shorter, bent, heavier. Sense how your arms hang. Turn your head left and right and notice the quality of

that movement. Sense the weight of your arms as they hang at your sides.

Now walk.

Sense how your arms swing. Are you aware of how your shoulder blades and collarbones participate in swinging your arms?

As you walk, look left and right. Sense how you turn your head and eyes. And notice the movement of your pelvis, how you turn with each step.

Compare how you feel and walk now with your normal patterns. What do you sense in yourself and how you move? Also, are you more aware of the room and everything around you?

PART SEVEN *Sitting*

1 Sit without leaning against the back of the chair, with your feet resting on the floor.

Turn your head right and left.

Notice how far and how easily you turn. Has there been any change from before? Recall choosing a point on the wall at the beginning of this lesson. Do you turn farther than that point now?

2 Close your eyes. Now, with your eyes closed, move your eyes left and right. Let that movement be as smooth and large as you can make it.

3 Let your head follow your eyes. As your eyes move toward the right, turn your head right. Then, as you look left, turn your head to the left.

Sense that movement in your eyes, your head, your neck, and along your spine.

4 Keep your eyes closed and have your shoulders join with your eyes and head. Your eyes, head, and shoulders all move together, harmoniously, left and right.

As you move your shoulders, rest your hands or forearms on your thighs somehow to support the weight of your arms. Your upper

Part Seven
Step One

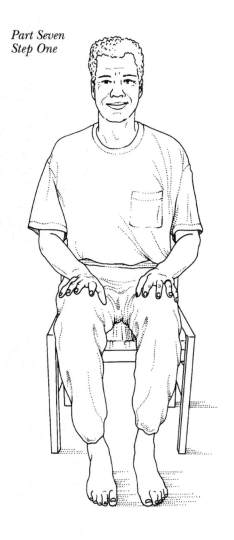

Part Seven
Step Four

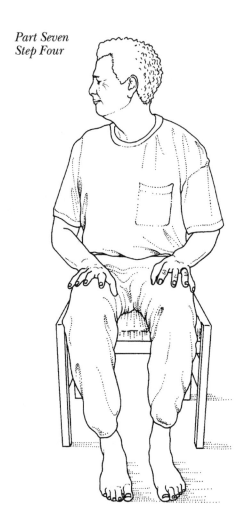

arms and elbows can move freely while your hands and forearms slide comfortably. If you like, you might also do this while holding your wrists or crossing your forearms. Then your arms can swing with your shoulders.

How far down your spine do you detect movement? Are you doing anything with your pelvis?

Part Seven
Step Five

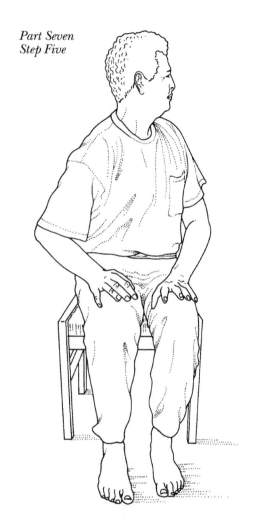

5 Intentionally add your pelvis to the turning movement. To turn your pelvis you have to move your legs. When your pelvis turns right, your left knee pushes forward and your right knee pulls back toward your pelvis. Your right knee pushes forward when you turn your pelvis left.

Turn your pelvis, shoulders, head, and eyes left and right. Do that a number of times, with your eyes closed.

Sense that movement everywhere, making it as free, smooth, and easy as you can.

6 As you turn left and right, gently open your eyes. Let your eyes move easily, without trying to see anything. Simply continue to turn smoothly from side to side.

Does having your eyes open affect the range or quality of turning? Are you less aware of yourself when your eyes are open? You may want to do a few movements with your eyes open and a few movements with your eyes closed, alternating to discover any differences.

When you sense that you are moving as easily with your eyes open as closed, begin to look at the walls and room around you. Can you actively look without disturbing the range or quality of the movement? What do you see?

Notice how far you are turning. Where is the point you chose on the wall now? Do you turn farther than you did a few moments ago? How much?

7 Sit easily. Do nothing. Rest. Be aware of how you are now, generally and compared with other times. How are you sitting? How are you breathing? Do you feel taller or straighter than before the lesson? Do you seem to be sitting with less effort?

If you were crossing the street and you heard a horn or the screech of brakes behind you, how would you turn? Do you think you could turn more quickly and easily with your shoulders and chest stiff, moving only your head and eyes? Or would you be safer if you turned more freely, with muscles everywhere participating? If you saw that you were in danger, how could you turn back most quickly to move to safety?

Each of us is capable of turning almost instantaneously, in any direction, even while walking or running. We can do that while keeping the eyes free to look forward or backward. That ability has to be innate, genetic, because if our ancestors had not been able to move that freely, they would not have survived to reproduce.

Even today, with our society that protects us when we are unaware, inflexible, or otherwise incapable, you are safer and healthier when you are aware and know how to move easily. We can be thankful for the advantages of civilization without becoming the victims of our own ignorance.

Gently, simply, move only your pelvis and sense how that involves everywhere above: your chest, back, shoulders, head, and eyes. Then move your head and look around, easily. Notice how free your shoulders are. Sense any movement in your chest, back, and pelvis. Even where you are not actively moving, you can be aware and eliminate any unnecessary effort or stiffening that might otherwise interfere.

8 Not now, but at another time, recall the differentiating movements you did lying on the floor. You can play with and explore the same movements and patterns while sitting, your eyes, head, shoulders, and pelvis, moving separately or together, singly or in pairs, in various combinations.

The differentiating/reintegrating process in this lesson applies to all learning. In various ways, you can see it in each of the lessons in this book. As I have said, we learn by sensing differences. Those differences that are useful, that somehow help us do what we want, can then be reintegrated into ongoing ways of acting and further exploring. The same process occurs in our most subtle or seemingly abstract activities, such as learning mathematics or a foreign language.

Leaning and Lifting

When we say something is three-dimensional, we acknowledge it as real and solid. Any three-dimensional object can be described in terms of three axes of rotation or six directions of movement, forward-backward, left-right, and up-down. In the first lesson, you were bending forward and backward in a way that involves rotating on a horizontal axis. The second lesson, turning and twisting, worked with rotating around a vertical axis. This lesson explores rotating around the third axis, sideways bending. In anatomy books, this is called lateral flexion.

In our everyday activities, almost everything we do involves simultaneously moving in all three directions. With regard to movements within the trunk, however, most people have the least awareness of sideways bending. Learning to bend sideways more easily will enhance your ability to turn or bend in all other directions. These movements also play an important, but usually unrecognized, role in sitting and walking, which we will explore in Lesson Five, *Effortless Sitting,* and Lesson Six, *Elegant Walking*.

In this lesson, you will be moving mostly on or toward one side to create clear differences. Conditioned by common systems of exercise, which almost always work both sides, some people want to immediately do everything symmetrically. You will learn the most if you restrain any such impulse and simply rest quietly at each interval. The final part of the lesson reintegrates your two sides. Later, in a few days perhaps, you may want to review this lesson while doing everything on the opposite side and moving in the opposite direction.

PART ONE   *Sitting*

1   Sit in your chair as you do normally. Sense how you are sitting.

Lean your head right and left. Your right ear goes toward your right shoulder, then your left ear goes toward your left shoulder. Do that simply, without turning, facing forward throughout the movement.

Notice what happens in your neck and elsewhere as you tilt your head this way. Sense any activity in your shoulders, your mid-back, and through your trunk into your pelvis. Does your weight shift on the chair as you lean your head to one side or to the other?

2   Sit forward from the back of the chair, with your feet flat on the floor.

Lift one sitting bone off the chair, lower it, then lift your other sitting bone. Tilt your pelvis left and right this way, from one side to the other.

Observe what you do as you tilt your pelvis. When either sitting bone lifts, sense how you shift your weight onto the opposite side. Notice how your head and shoulders move. As always, keep the movement small enough so that you are really comfortable. Breathe freely.

Pause for a moment.

3   Again, simply lean your head left and right. Move your right ear toward your right shoulder, then your left ear toward your left shoulder. Face forward.

Can you now sense how your weight shifts on the chair, that you move your pelvis as you tilt your head? You *are* moving your pelvis; the question is whether you are aware.

4   Bring your right arm over the top of your head and place your right hand on your left ear. Hold your head with your arm as securely as comfortable, your upper arm touching or close to

your right ear. Your left arm can remain wherever it is most comfortable, perhaps with the hand or forearm resting on your thigh.

Move your right arm and head together, as a unit, to the right and back to the middle. As your head and arm move to the right, your right elbow goes toward the floor. Face forward throughout the movement.

Notice how your head moves now, with your arm in this position, compared with a moment ago when you were simply tilting your head. Does your head move farther this way? Are you more aware of your right side, chest, and back? Did one side of your pelvis lift, shifting your weight, as you moved toward the right?

To answer these questions, do this movement a number of times.

Lower your arm and rest briefly.

5 Again, raise your right arm and hold your head as before, with your right hand on your left ear.

While holding your head in this way, lift your left sitting bone off the chair as you move your head and arm toward the right. Lower your left sitting bone and sit evenly as you move your head back to the center. Do this a number of times, lifting the left side of your pelvis to lean to the right, then return to the center.

Notice how far you move your head now, and how easily. Sense how this movement involves your ribs, chest, and back.

Pause.

6 Now lift your right sitting bone while simultaneously moving your head and arm to the right. Lower the right side of your pelvis and sit evenly as you move your head and arm back to the center.

If you were watching yourself in a mirror, you would see your spine curving like a C. Your right elbow and the right side of your pelvis move toward each other and away from each other. Close your eyes if that helps you to be more aware of how you are moving. Do the movement 15 or 20 times, easily.

Sense how far and how easily you move your head while tilting your pelvis in this way. What happens in your ribs and throughout your right side as you bend sideways and then straighten?

Part One
Step Four

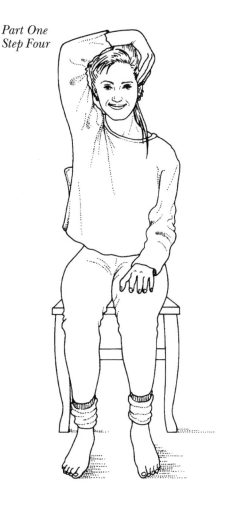

Part One
Step Six

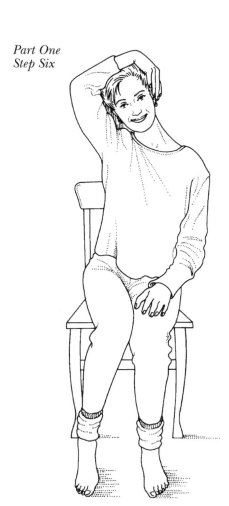

Rest for a moment, lowering your arm if you like.

7 Again, lift your right arm and place it over the top of your head, with your right hand on or near your left ear.

Move your head and arm toward the right and back to the center 3 or 4 times while lifting the right side of your pelvis. Then do 3 or 4 movements with your head and arm toward the right while you lift your left sitting bone. Repeat these movements, changing the movement in your pelvis after each 3 or 4 repetitions.

Sense how these variations involve differences in your ribs and throughout your right side. Notice how far your head moves in each case. As always, remember to breathe freely, neither forcing nor inhibiting, so that your ribs can move easily.

Lower your arm and rest.

8 Tilt your head right and left, simply. Leave both arms at your sides, or resting comfortably on your thighs.

How does this movement compare with when you did it a few minutes ago? Does your head tilt more easily toward the right? Sense anything you might be doing differently in your neck, shoulder, ribs, back, pelvis.

9 Rest. Sit easily. Compare how you are sitting now with how you sat at the beginning of this lesson.

After doing these movements mostly to the right, can you detect any differences between your two sides? Does one side feel larger, lighter, more alive? Do you seem to be breathing more on one side? Without judging what is better or habitual, simply be aware.

PART TWO *Lying on Your Back*

1 Lie on your back and rest. Sense how you contact the floor now. Especially, compare your right side and your left. Is there any difference in your shoulder blades? What about your pelvis and hip joints—do you rest more securely on one side than on the other side?

When aware, most people detect differences between the two sides. This is quite reasonable, since almost everyone favors one hand or side for many actions, such as writing or eating. Some people are obviously asymmetrical. In many tennis players, for example, the arm that holds the racket is often noticeably more developed than the other arm, with corresponding changes throughout the shoulder and back.

Imagine a picture of yourself, taken from within, that shows your skeleton and muscles and the surface of your skin all around. Examine the clarity and accuracy of that picture, the details. Some areas may be easy to picture in this way, while other places remain dark or vague. One side may be larger, brighter, or better

Part Two
Step One

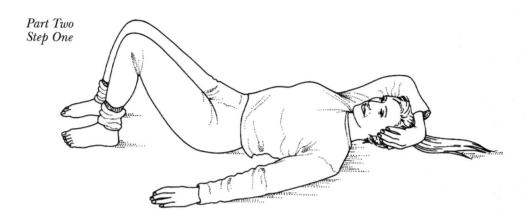

defined than the other. This way of imaging can be an extremely effective aid to learning, and I encourage you to take time, now and in the future, to develop this.

2 Bend your legs so your feet are flat on the floor. Bring your right arm over the top of your head and place your right hand on your left ear in the same way you did while sitting. Hold your head as securely as comfortable. Place your right forearm in contact with the very top of your head, not on your forehead. Your right upper arm is near your right ear, or even touches it. Leave your left arm comfortably at your side.

Move your head with your right arm toward the right and back to the middle. Keep your face toward the ceiling so that the back of your head slides on the floor. Use your arm to do the work—you can pull your head to the right with your hand, and push with your upper arm to move your head back to the middle.

This is the same movement you were doing while sitting. Yet you have changed your orientation to space and gravity, which alters this action in fundamental ways. Sense what you are doing in your right shoulder, your chest, your back, and all along your right side. What differences do you detect in the range and quality of movement now compared with when you were sitting?

Do this a number of times, to sense clearly what you are doing.

Pause. Lower your arm to your side.

Part Three
Step One

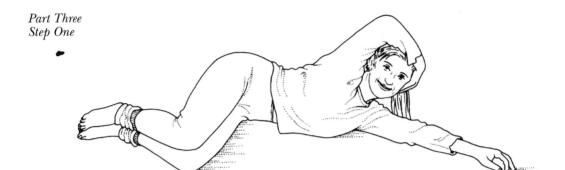

3 Rest. Lie still. Do nothing. Again, notice how you contact the floor and how you picture yourself. Compare your right and left sides, your neck, shoulders, and back with before. Is there any change?

PART THREE   *On Your Left Side*

1 Roll to lie on your left side. Rest your head on or near your left arm, with your left arm bent or straight, as you prefer. If it makes you more comfortable, use a small pad or pillow to help support your head, instead of your arm or along with it. Bend your legs so there is approximately a 90-degree angle at your knees, with your hip joints bent somewhere between 45 and 60 degrees. Bending your legs helps you be more stable and comfortable than if you keep your legs straight.

Bring your right arm over the top of your head and place your right hand on your left ear.

Move your head and arm toward the right and back to the middle. This now means lifting your head toward the ceiling and lowering your head again. Each time you lower your head, fully release any effort before lifting again. As always, do this movement simply, keeping it small enough so you are comfortable.

Once again, you are doing the same movement while the world has shifted position. How does this change in your orientation affect the range and quality of the movement? What do you notice from the changing pull of gravity? Compare the friction

Part Three
Step Two

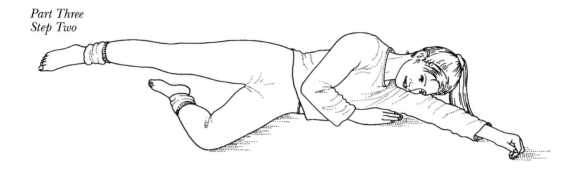

and pressure of the floor on your left side with before, when you were on your back.

Do 15 or 20 movements and sense what happens in your neck and shoulder, ribs, chest, back—all along your right side. Can you detect any movement in your pelvis?

Roll onto your back and rest for a few moments.

2 Again, lie on your left side with your head on your left arm or a pillow. As a moment ago, bend your left leg at the knee and hip joint. Extend your right leg so it is in line with your trunk.

Lift your straight right leg toward the ceiling, and lower it, keeping your leg in line with your trunk. In this position, lifting your leg toward the ceiling means moving it to the right. Each time you lower your leg, let it rest on the floor for an instant and sense the weight of your foot on the floor as the muscles let go.

Remember, the less you do, the more you can sense and learn. While various systems of calisthenics use sideways leg-lifts to tone the thighs, waist, and hip area, we are interested in enhancing awareness. Only lift your leg as high as it goes easily, perhaps just a few inches. Each time you lift your leg, see if you can use less effort. Repeat this 10 or 15 times.

Notice what happens in your right hip joint and in your pelvis. Can you sense movement further up your right side, in your ribs, chest, and back? What else are you aware of?

Pause. If you like, briefly roll onto your back and rest. Then lie on your side again.

Part Three
Step Three

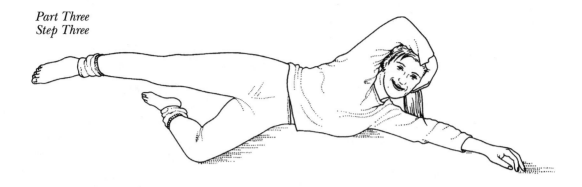

3 Raise your right arm and hold your head as before, your arm over the top of your head and your right hand on your left ear.

Now, simultaneously, lift your head with your arm and lift your right leg. Lift and lower your head and leg together. Remember to sense your weight on the floor for an instant each time you lower your leg and head.

Is it twice as much work to lift your head and leg together as lifting one or the other? Why not? Do your head and leg each lift higher now, together, than when you were lifting either one by itself?

Lift and lower your head and leg together many times as you seek to answer these questions. Sense where and how you are moving all along your right side—your hip joint, pelvis, ribs, back, shoulder, everywhere. Remember, any time you are holding or forcing your breath, the ribs and trunk cannot move freely. See if you can find a way to breathe that assists you with lifting and lowering your head and leg.

Pause briefly.

4 Now, again, move only your head and arm. As before, lift and lower your head with your right arm. Leave your right leg extended or bent, in contact with your left leg or the floor.

Has this movement become any easier or larger than before? Notice how moving your head and arm involves your whole right side, all the way down to and including your pelvis and hip joint. Can you detect that?

5 Observe how you are breathing as you lift and lower your head. Is there some pattern? Were you coordinating your breathing with the movement even without being specifically instructed to do so?

Do that deliberately. Breathe out as you lift your head and in as you lower. Each time you lower, pause for an instant before you lift again. Let your breathing regulate the height and rate of the movement.

Now reverse the pattern of breathing. Breathe in as you lift your head and out as you lower. Do the movement this way a number of times.

Reverse the pattern again. Do 2 or 3 movements, breathing out as you lift. Then do 2 or 3 movements breathing in as you lift.

Sense the differences in these two ways of lifting your head. Which way of breathing allows you to lift higher, more easily? Discover all you can about these differences.

Notice what happens in your ribs all along your right side.

Roll onto your back and rest. Lie still and do nothing for a moment. Breathe easily and sense how you are now.

PART FOUR *Lying on Your Back*

1 Bend your legs so your feet are flat on the floor. Bring your right arm over the top of your head and place your right hand on or near your left ear.

Once again, move your head with your arm toward the right and back to the middle.

Has this movement become easier or larger as a result of what you were doing while on your side? Sense the movement all through your right side, in your head and neck, your shoulder, shoulder blade and collarbone, along your spine, and all your ribs. Notice when and how the ribs squeeze together, and when they move apart.

Are you more aware now? Can you detect any activity in your hip joint and pelvis?

89

Part Four
Step One

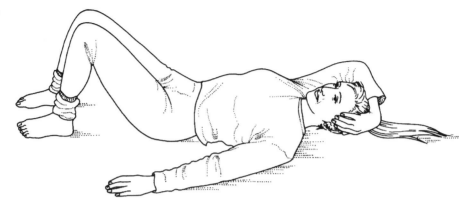

Do this movement 15 or 20 times, easily, comparing the range and quality of this movement with when you did it before.

Rest. Bring both arms to your sides.

2 Compare your right side, where you have been doing all the work, and your left. What differences do you sense between your two sides? Which side feels more in contact with the floor? Does one side feel lighter, longer, more alive? On your right side, do you feel tired and heavy from working?

Recall that learning involves perceiving differences, most commonly distinguishing between before and after or between left and right. We are all accustomed to exercise techniques and therapies that work symmetrically, yet doing so may not be conducive to sensing differences and learning.

Rest for a few more moments as you continue to sense any differences. If you seem somewhat unbalanced, good. Simply be aware of that. If you feel a desire to wiggle or stretch, see if you can remain still. Wiggling or stretching will obscure any subtle changes and interfere with your learning. Allow time to notice any differences, between your two sides, and relative to when you began this lesson.

3 Slowly roll to one side and stand. Notice toward which side you rolled. Did you roll out of habit, toward the side you usually

choose? Or did your rolling somehow relate to any differences you sensed between the two sides?

4 Stand for a moment. Can you sense a difference between the two sides while standing? Do you seem heavier on one side? Might you be leaning to one side?

5 Begin to walk, slowly. Does one leg seem to take a longer stride? Do your arms swing differently?

If you walked with your eyes closed, would you follow a straight line, or veer off toward one side? Which one?

Allow yourself enough time to be aware of any differences between your right and left sides as you stand and walk. Some people become aware only gradually, and you may want to allow five or ten minutes for this exploring.

PART FIVE *Integrating the Left Side*

Some Awareness Through Movement lessons work with one side only, often for much longer than we have been doing. In an extended workshop or training program, I might do a lesson like that before a break for lunch or at the end of the day, encouraging people to sense any differences when they return to their everyday activities.

In doing that, something very interesting and significant occurs: in many cases, benefits or improvements are spontaneously transferred from one side to the other. While this spontaneous integration may seem surprising, even miraculous, it is really an everyday miracle. It is natural for us to favor and adopt more effective ways of functioning. If we did not, human development and evolution could not occur. This is how babies learn to crawl, walk, and talk. Moshe's ability to understand and apply this insight is a key reason for the success of the Feldenkrais Method.

Another way to integrate the two sides would be to simply repeat the movements taught in the preceding section on the left side. Now we are going to integrate the two sides in a third way.

1   Lie on your back. Bend your legs so your feet are flat on the floor. Once again bring your right arm over the top of your head to place your right hand on or near your left ear.

Move your head with your arm toward the right and back to the middle as you have been doing.

Now notice how your left side participates in this movement. What happens in your ribs on the left as you move toward the right and back? Can you sense any movement in your left shoulder blade and/or change in how your arm contacts the floor? Are you moving at all in your pelvis on the left side, or in that hip joint?

Be aware how moving to the right involves all of yourself. You have been moving on both sides all along, although until now your left side has been mostly passive. As you continue to move your head to the right and back to the middle, shift your attention from place to place to become more aware everywhere. As I have suggested in previous lessons, a good way to do this is to sense or picture your skeleton, bones and joints, and your entire surface, your skin.

Lower your right arm. Rest briefly.

2   Bring your left arm over the top of your head and place your left hand on your right ear.

Now, in your imagination only, move your head and arm toward the left and back to the center. Do not actually move; only imagine doing so.

To imagine, some people construct a picture and see themselves doing the movement. A more effective alternative is to re-create the various sensations of muscles contracting or lengthening, friction with the floor, your clothes, and the air around you. Make this imagined movement as vivid, accurate, and detailed as you can. Recall what you experienced a moment ago while doing the movement toward the right and use that to provide more detail regarding what occurs on your left.

Be aware of your breathing as you do this. When moving your head and arm to the right, you found ways to breathe freely and assist the movement. As you imagine moving to the left, breathe as easily. Many people hold their breath when studying or concentrating in any way, and this seems to be characteristic of people who have difficulty being attentive, especially children in school.

While breathing easily, imagine moving your head to the left a few more times.

3 Rest. Lower your left arm. Rest is just as important after imagining the movement as after actually doing it. Research has shown that imagined movement completes neurological connections and sends messages to the muscles similar to when one actually moves. In fact, fatigue occurs in the nervous system before it occurs in the muscles; we normally do not recognize that, however, because we are not sufficiently aware.

4 Roll to lie on your right side. Bend your legs as you did earlier while lying on your left side.

Bring your left arm over the top of your head and place your left hand on your right ear.

Now imagine lifting your head with your left arm. Do nothing, only imagine. Once again, recall all that you experienced while doing the movement on the right. The awareness you gained doing the movement toward the right will help you accurately imagine doing this to the left, and imagining accurately helps you benefit and learn.

Again, and always, breathe freely as you do this. Can you recall a preferred way to coordinate your breathing with the movement?

Picture, imagine, and sense how every part of you would move if you were actually lifting and lowering your head with your left arm. Sense your ribs all around, in your sides, chest, and back. See how detailed you can make the movement in your imagination.

Pause for a moment.

5 Straighten your left leg, or simply imagine doing so. Now imagine lifting your leg. Do that a number of times, breathing freely.

Each time you imagine your leg returning to the floor, sense the weight of your left foot and leg contacting the floor or right leg.

As you imagine lifting and lowering, sense the movement in your hip joints, pelvis, ribs, and all along your spine.

6 Imagine lifting your leg and your head and arm at the same time.

As you do that, imagine the movement in both sides. Imagine how your ribs move, when and how they squeeze together or fan apart. Sense how your right side presses the floor differently as you imagine lifting and lowering on the left. Be aware of breathing easily as you sense or imagine the movement everywhere.

Imagine the movement a number of times. Then roll onto your back and rest.

7 While lying on your back, bring your left arm over the top of your head and place your hand on or near your right ear. Or, if you choose, simply imagine doing this.

Once again, imagine moving your head with your left arm toward the left and back to the center. Remember to breathe in the way that best assists you with this movement.

Sense and imagine the movement on both sides, your hip joints, pelvis, ribs, shoulders, neck, and head. As you imagine, see if you can discover ways for your right side to assist actively in doing this movement toward the left.

Imagine a few more movements, making these as large and free and easy as possible.

8 Rest. Extend your legs. Lie still, with both arms at your sides. Sense how you are now.

Do you notice any change in how you contact the floor from a few minutes ago, after doing the movements only toward the right side? How does your contact on both sides compare with when you began this lesson?

Picture yourself, your skeleton and the surface of your skin, and notice any changes from before. Compare your left and right, and both sides with before the lesson. Can you picture yourself more clearly, with more detail? Are there places that seem brighter and more vivid? If you picture yourself in colors, have those changed?

When I teach this lesson, we sometimes do the movements to one side for thirty or forty minutes. Then we imagine moving to the other side for only five or ten minutes. Some people report that they learn and experience more changes on the left side after only imagining the movements than they did on the right side while actually doing them. Is that true for you? An explanation for this is that we commonly use more effort than necessary to do a movement; while imagining we are generally more relaxed and comfortable, and therefore better able to learn.

9 Slowly roll to either side and stand. Did you roll toward the same side as when you stood a few minutes ago, or did you roll toward the opposite side? As always, there is no right or wrong with this.

PART SIX *Sitting*

1 Sit forward on your chair, with your feet on the floor. Begin to simply tilt your pelvis left and right. Lift one sitting bone and then the other to lean right and left.

Let your head and shoulders move toward the left as you lift your right sitting bone. Your head and shoulders move toward the right as you lift your left sitting bone. This means that your spine is more or less straight throughout the movement.

Sense the movement all through your spine, in your ribs on both sides, and everywhere as you do that. Notice what happens in your legs, how your thighs move slightly. Leave your feet and lower legs relaxed and balanced.

Pause.

2 Now move your pelvis in the same way, lifting one sitting bone then the other, while curving your spine like a C. As your spine curves, your head tilts yet stays over your pelvis.

Imagine looking at yourself from in front or behind, and see if you can do the movement so that your spine makes a continuous, smooth C curve from the top of your head to the tip of your tail.

Sense the movement all along your spine and in your ribs all around on both sides. Notice where and how the ribs fan apart, and where and how they squeeze together.

Part Six
Step One

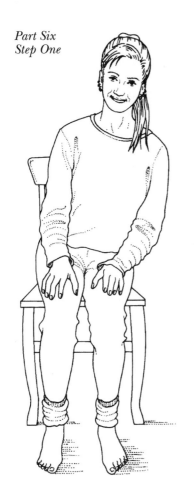

Part Six
Step Two

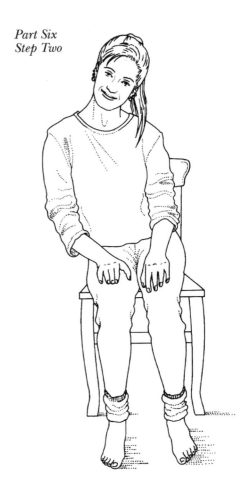

Compare how you lift your pelvis when your spine curves like a C with how you lift your pelvis when keeping your spine straight. Which way of moving allows you to lift one side of your pelvis higher, with less effort? Which feels more comfortable? Easier?

Rest for a moment.

3 Bring your left arm over the top of your head and place your left hand on your right ear. Move your head and arm together toward

Part Six
Step Three

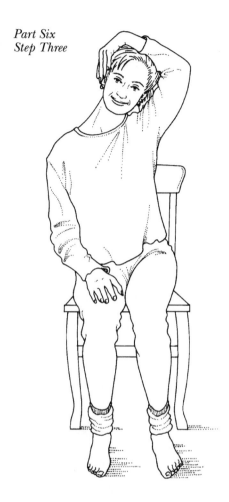

the left and back to the center, your elbow moving toward the floor on your left each time.

Do this a number of times, simply.

Each time you move your head and arm toward the left, sense which sitting bone could lift more easily. Would you move your head and arm farther and more comfortably while lifting your left sitting bone or your right? Experiment and find which is easier.

Find the easier way and continue to lean and lift, 10 or 15 times. Make the movement as large as comfortable. Breathe freely. Be aware of your ribs and the movement all around and through your trunk.

Lower your arm. Briefly rest.

4 Bring your right arm over the top of your head and place your right hand on or near your left ear. Move your head and arm together toward the right and back to the center.

Compare how you do this movement now with how you did it in the first part of this lesson. Is it easier now? Does your head move farther, with less effort? Sense the movement all through your back, in your ribs all around, and down into your pelvis and hip joints.

Lower your arm and rest for a moment.

5 Once again, sit forward on your chair, with your feet on the floor. Tilt your pelvis left and right, lifting first one sitting bone and then the other. Lean right and left.

Do that a few times, keeping your spine straight. Then do several movements while curving your spine like a C. Sense how far and how easily you lift your pelvis and lean toward each side.

Continue to alternate those variations after each 3 or 4 movements, your spine either remaining straight or curving like a C.

Make the movements smoother, larger, easier. See if you can eliminate any unnecessary effort.

Briefly rest.

6 Begin to tilt your pelvis left and right while keeping your head more or less in the middle. Your head can be mostly still, as if you were looking at someone or something.

Gradually lift either side of your pelvis further, while keeping your head in relatively the same place, although tilting slightly. Be sure you do not stiffen, in your neck or anywhere.

Breathe easily. Observe whether you coordinate your breathing with the movement in any way. Can you find a way to breathe that assists with lifting and lowering your pelvis?

How far do you move your pelvis now? Sense the movement all through your trunk. Notice what happens in your ribs all around. Compare your left and right sides, where your ribs squeeze together and where they fan apart.

Let your head move more freely and make the movement as large as you can. Do whatever you can, comfortably, to make this movement larger and easier.

Sense the movement all through your trunk, in your spine from your pelvis through to your head, in your ribs all around, in your shoulder blades and collarbones.

7 Gradually make the movement smaller, until you are lifting your pelvis to lean left and right with such delicacy that someone watching you would not notice. You slightly lift one sitting bone, then the other, to make a very small movement of tilting your pelvis.

Notice how you are sitting as you do this. Are you comfortable? Can you sit easily this way, even without leaning against the back of the chair? Sense your head, neck, shoulders, and back. Observe how your weight is supported by your pelvis as you do this very small movement.

8 Rest. Sit easily for a moment. Lean against the back of the chair if you like.

Slowly stand. And walk. Notice how your weight shifts from side to side. Sense that movement in your pelvis, all through your spine, in your ribs, in your head and shoulders.

Are you aware of any differences from your usual way of walking? Especially be attentive to how you shift your weight from one leg to the other. Do you do anything with your pelvis?

Posture and "Acture"

Good posture concerns most people, yet we rarely think about what this means other than "standing up straight." Moshe noted that the root of *posture* is *post,* which describes something fixed, static, rigid. He coined the term *acture* to suggest the way the spine dynamically aligns and realigns with every action. As he defined it, *acture* describes the way someone sits or stands when not engaging in any intentional act, the neutral position to which one returns after enacting some intention. Good "acture" is that which enables one to act spontaneously with the greatest degree of freedom. These ideas provide an excellent, functional definition for truly good posture.

Scoliosis is the medical term for an abnormal sideways curve or twist in the spine. Medical literature describes most cases of scoliosis as "idiopathic," meaning that the cause is not understood. What is well known, however, is that the most serious and troubling cases of scoliosis occur in adolescent girls. Someone with a severe scoliosis may have a hunched back, compressed lungs and internal organs, and a variety of serious health problems. Standard treatments include exercise or physical therapy, chiropractic adjustments, or rigid braces that may need to be worn every night or all day, sometimes for years. Research has not proved any of these treatments effective, however. In serious cases of scoliosis, surgeons install a rigid metal rod or use wires to straighten and reinforce the spine.

Like most people, I recall my mother telling me to stand up straight when I was young, and I occasionally hear parents command their children to do that. Children usually straighten

A few years ago, Conrad and Phyllis, a couple in their late sixties or early seventies, attended a six-week class in which I taught the lessons in this book. They stopped by my office several weeks after the final class to thank me and tell me of their experience:

Their son lives near San Francisco, a six-hour drive north from Santa Barbara. For many years, driving to visit him had been unpleasant. Conrad and Phyllis would occasionally have to stop and get out of the car to stretch, and would arrive feeling stiff and tired. When they made the trip the previous weekend, however, they had reminded each other to be aware of how they were sitting in the car. While driving, Conrad and Phyllis had done the movements they learned in my class. In this way, they told me, they had been able to drive straight through to their son's house, and when they got out of the car they felt as comfortable as they normally did after only a short trip.

Many people report similar benefits, and I am always pleased when my students discover their own ways to apply what they are learning. As Conrad and Phyllis learned, straining and stiffening are only habits. When aware, you can find more comfortable and effective ways to do whatever you like.

for a while, as I did, but after a short time the effort required becomes unpleasant, or attention wanders, and the more comfortable and familiar "posture" is resumed. If willpower were the answer, no one would have bad posture. Moshe used to tell a detailed and colorful true story of a stoop-shouldered 70-year-old man whose 95-year-old mother had been telling him to stand up straight since he was a young boy. Neither the man nor his mother knew how to alter the pattern.

Instead of trying to correct bad posture or scoliosis by imposing some arbitrary idea of how the spine should be, the Feldenkrais Method helps people learn to move more freely and improve their "acture." In the preceding lesson, you learned how to curve your spine to create a C curve scoliosis. But while someone with a diagnosed scoliosis does that to one side only, compulsively, you learned to curve toward either side, voluntarily. You could also learn to make an S curve scoliosis or other variations. When you can curve or twist your spine in many different ways, you can also be symmetrical and balanced.

The six lessons in this book can be extremely helpful for preventing or treating scoliosis and other postural disorders. If you have any concerns or difficulties, do the lessons carefully, moving only within the small range that is both symmetrical and comfortable. Individual Feldenkrais lessons can greatly facilitate your progress.

Moshe recognized that, when freed from habitual constraints and inhibitions, we spontaneously favor positions and ways of moving that are functional and symmetrical. You can clearly see that in young children. As you become more aware and learn to move more comfortably, you may confirm it through your experience.

I can tell many stories of people who have had a scoliosis reverse, at least partially, and I have never seen anyone fail to improve. Doctors and medical scientists say that these anecdotal accounts do not prove anything, however, and I agree. One day, soon I hope, independent researchers will examine the Feldenkrais Method and incorporate these six lessons or others into their research protocols. The Feldenkrais Approach to scoliosis is so simple and understandable that it seems reasonable to use it before more strenuous or invasive approaches. I am confident it will continue to bring good results.

Uninhibited Breathing

For a few moments, simply be aware of how you are breathing. See if you can do that without interfering or changing anything.

Sense the air passing through your nose and sinuses. Does the air pass smoothly, or can you detect any obstruction or turbulence? Are you aware of the air passing outward as well as inward?

Notice how you are moving to breathe. Do you sense movement in your chest, your abdomen, or both? Are you aware of any movement in your sides and back? What about your shoulders— can you detect any rising and falling? Do you sense clearly and easily, or are there places where you are not sure if you are moving? Also, notice any external cues to how you are moving, the weight, friction, or rustle of your clothing, or changes in how you contact your chair or any other surface.

When I talk with people about breathing, many express concerns or describe difficulties. While only some experience asthma or other severe problems, a majority say that they often hold their breath, at least partially, and almost everyone occasionally yawns, sighs, or otherwise pauses. Smokers seem generally to breathe shallowly, except when smoking, as if they only know how to breathe fully with the cigarette to remind them.

Stress and stress-related difficulties always involve some distur- bance of breathing. Various psychological and spiritual practices, including yoga and some types of biofeedback, work with breathing to relieve stress. I know a number of teachers or therapists who like to tell their friends and students to "Breathe!" When I am nearby, I like to observe how people respond to that command. Most immediately breathe in, typically in an exaggerated way. I like to do the opposite, intentionally breathing out slowly and completely. On a few occasions, the person who said "Breathe!" noticed me and became confused or annoyed, which I found quite amusing.

Inhaling is only part of breathing. In focusing on the inhalation and ignoring the exhalation, which most people seem to do, the overall process is disturbed. If you had a glass that was half full of water and you wanted to pour in as much water as possible, you would empty it first. In the same way, you will breathe in more easily after breathing out fully. In fact, the primary way breathing is regulated neurologically is based on eliminating carbon dioxide; the need to take in more oxygen is secondary.

This lesson explores the movements involved in breathing. As you breathe in, the diaphragm and other muscles which attach to the ribs pull in one direction to make the internal space larger. Air then enters to fill that space. To breathe out, opposing muscles compress that internal space. In each of the first three lessons, you discovered how breathing more easily can assist you in moving your head, trunk, arms, and legs. This lesson emphasizes movements within the trunk.

The movements in this lesson are smaller and somewhat more subtle than those in the three previous lessons. Some people fall asleep while breathing slowly and attentively with this lesson; if you do sleep, simply resume when you awaken. Continue with each step in the lesson for several minutes, as long as you remain actively interested and learning.

PART ONE *Lying on Your Back*

1 Lie on the floor with your arms at your sides. Your legs can be extended or bent, however you are more comfortable.

Breathe easily and sense how you are breathing now. Simply

notice where and how you move as you breathe. Observe your breathing without doing anything more.

2 Rest either hand on your lower abdomen, below the navel. Begin to breathe so that your hand rises as you breathe in and lowers as you breathe out. Deliberately breathe in a way that makes the movement in your lower abdomen as large as possible in both directions.

Your hand is there to help you sense the movement, nothing more. And do not tilt your pelvis. Simply expand and contract your lower abdomen with your breath.

Pushing the belly forward fully is difficult for many people. We live in a culture that thinks a tight, firm abdomen is youthful and sexy, and some people spend a great deal of time and money to strengthen their "abs." To try always to hold muscles tight, however, leads to fatigue and weakness, which is one reason people often become potbellied and flabby when they stop exercising. More important, holding the abdominal muscles tighter than necessary generally restricts breathing and moving. If you learn to push your belly forward more freely, you will tone those muscles and naturally be more lean and attractive.

See how large a movement you can make in your abdomen in both directions, slowly. Do this for several minutes. This is often called abdominal or diaphragmatic breathing. Some people believe that we should always breathe this way.

Be attentive to your comfort as you do this. If you breathe too strongly or quickly you may hyperventilate, which is not what this lesson is teaching.

Pause. Breathe easily, without thought or effort.

3 Now place one hand on your upper chest, above the nipples. Breathe in a way that makes the movement there as large as possible. See how much you can expand and lift your chest while you breathe in. Then squeeze to compress your chest as you breathe out. As long as you are comfortable, make that movement as large as possible.

If your sinuses are at all blocked you can breathe through your mouth as well as your nose, at least on the out breath. All animals

Part One
Step Four

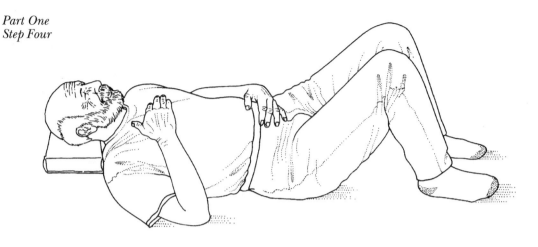

breathe through mouth and nose, except human beings who have been taught that breathing with the mouth open is unhealthy, improper, or unattractive. Breathing freely, it seems to me, is more important than looking good.

Sense the movement in your upper chest in both directions, expanding and contracting. Stay with this and explore the range of movement in your upper chest for several minutes.

Some people believe that this is correct, healthy breathing.

Rest briefly. Again, breathe easily without thinking about how.

4 Place one hand on your upper chest and one hand on your lower abdomen.

Take a moderate breath, not deep, and hold your breath for a few moments. While holding that breath, squeeze the muscles in your upper chest to push the air into your lower abdomen, then squeeze the lower abdomen to push the air into your upper chest. This means that one hand will rise while the other falls, alternating like a seesaw.

To help you understand and do this, picture a balloon, partially inflated and tied. When you squeeze either end of the balloon, you force the air to the opposite end. With this movement, your trunk is the balloon and you provide the knot by holding your

105

breath. You squeeze your upper chest to force the air to your belly, then the reverse.

Do that 3 or 4 times. Then breathe out and pause for a moment as you breathe easily once or twice. When you are ready, breathe in, hold your breath, and repeat the movement. Be attentive to your comfort.

Play with this seesaw movement. Make it larger and stronger or lighter and quicker, comfortably. See how many times you can seesaw before pausing to breathe. Also, while holding your breath helps you learn and understand, you might find ways to do this seesaw movement while breathing easily, in and out.

To the best of my knowledge, no one believes that this is the correct way to breathe. It is, however, an excellent way to learn to be more aware of how you move your chest and abdomen.

Rest for a few moments. Breathe easily.

5 Again, breathe with your upper chest mostly. Rest one hand there if that helps you sense how you are moving.

Has this become larger or easier as a result of playing with the seesaw movement? See how large you can make the movement, both the expansion and the contraction.

6 Now breathe so that the movement is as large as you can make it in your lower abdomen.

Notice if this has become easier, or better defined. How large can you make this movement now? Sense how the movement involves the lowest part of your abdomen, down to your pubic bone.

7 Rest. Breathe simply and easily for a few moments. Notice how you breathe spontaneously.

PART TWO *Lying on Your Front*

1 Roll to lie on your front, and turn your head toward either side. Whichever way your head is facing, bring that arm up, so that you can look at it. Leave the other arm at your side. If you find it awkward to lie on your front, use pillows under your chest or abdomen to make yourself comfortable. Remember, comfort is essential for learning.

Part Two
Step Two

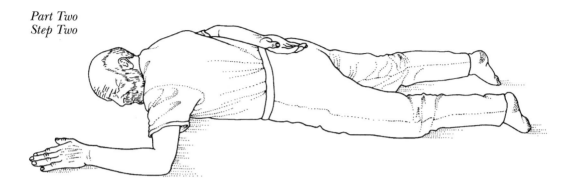

2 Breathe with your lower abdomen, as you were just doing while lying on your back. Expand and contract your lower abdomen as fully as you can.

Notice how lying on your front, with your belly against the floor, changes the range and quality of the movement. Compare how you now expand and contract your abdomen with the same movement when lying on your back.

Do you sense your lower back lifting and lowering with each breath?

Take the arm that is at your side and rest the back of that hand on your lower back. With your hand, sense how your lower back lifts toward the ceiling as you breathe in and lowers toward the floor as you breathe out.

Do what you can, comfortably, to make the movement in your lower back larger. See if you can do that with your breathing, not by tilting your pelvis.

We mostly think about breathing in front, primarily because we see the front. But the ribs attach to the spine and the diaphragm anchors into the spine and pelvis. It is impossible to move in front without doing something in back. You are three-dimensional. Learning to sense how breathing involves movement in your back as well as in front will help you breathe more freely and do any movement more easily. In addition, as you learn to breathe and move the back muscles more freely, you will be better able to relieve any stiffness or tightness there.

3 Turn your head to the other side. On the side you are now facing, bring your arm up so you can see it, with the other arm resting on the floor at your side.

Now breathe to expand and contract your upper chest. Make the movement in your upper chest as large as comfortable in both directions.

Once again, the floor prevents forward movement while gravity pulls you downward. Can you sense how this movement occurs in your upper back?

The area between the shoulder blades is vague and undefined for most people, and it may be difficult for you to sense movement there at first. Simply imagine how your upper back lifts as you breathe in and lowers as you breathe out. You will soon begin to sense how your shoulder blades move to accommodate the lifting and lowering in your spine.

Some people can comfortably reach with their hand to touch the area between the shoulder blades, either from above or from below. If you want to, and you can do so easily, touch that area with your fingers.

Whether you sense it or not, you are moving your upper back, your ribs, your spine, and your shoulder blades. As always, the more you sense and become aware, the more freely and easily you can move.

Picture this movement as clearly as you can. Does your back move straight upward as you breathe in and downward as you breathe out? Or does the movement occur at various angles in accordance with the curve of your spine? Sense whatever you can as you breathe in ways that mobilize your upper back fully and comfortably.

4 Roll to lie on your back. Rest. Breathe easily and sense how you are now.

PART THREE   *Lying on Your Back*

1 Bend your legs so your feet are flat on the floor. Once again, breathe in a way that expands and contracts your upper chest as fully as comfortable.

As you sense the movement in your chest, also notice how your upper back presses against the floor. Sense the changing pressure and contact as you breathe in and out.

Does sensing your back help you breathe more easily, so that your chest lifts and lowers more freely? See how large you can make that movement, both expanding and contracting.

Pause.

2 Now breathe while emphasizing the movement in your lower abdomen. Expand and contract there as fully as you can comfortably.

As you breathe, can you sense the changing pressure of your lower back against the floor? Do you seem to be breathing more freely or easily than when you were on your back before? What are you aware of now?

Make the movement as large as possible, expanding and contracting. See how far down into your pelvis you can sense the movement.

Rest briefly. Breathe easily, spontaneously.

3 Gradually find a way to expand your lower abdomen as you breathe out. Do this without tilting your pelvis. Breathe in easily, without expanding in your abdomen. Then push the lowest area of your belly forward, toward the ceiling, as you breathe out.

This is the reverse of what you have been doing until now. For obvious reasons, this is sometimes called paradoxical or reverse breathing. You may want to rest one or both hands on your lower abdomen to help you sense the movement. Use your abdominal muscles as fully as you can to make this movement as large as comfortable.

Sense this movement in the lowest area of your pelvis, below the navel and into the pubic bone. Notice if there is anything happening in your lower back, any change in how you press or contact the floor.

Believe it or not, there are people who teach that this is a correct, healthy way to breathe, at least under certain circumstances. If you learn to do this skillfully, you may begin to understand why.

4 Rest for a moment. Breathe easily without thought or effort. Sense how you breathe now. Has there been any change from when you began this lesson? What are you aware of?

5 Place one hand on your lower abdomen and one hand on your upper chest. Breathe so both hands lift as you breathe in and lower as you breathe out.

Sense the movement above and below, in and out, all together. Do that slowly, easily, comfortably.

Move your hands to touch your chest and abdomen in different places as you continue to breathe this way. See if you can discover the movement in each rib, in your sides as well as in front, even under the armpits and in the collarbones. And sense the movement all the way down into the deepest part of your pelvis, under your pubic bone.

Do this for several minutes as you explore the movement everywhere.

6 Rest. Extend your legs. Let your arms be at your sides. Breathe normally, whatever that means to you now.

Be aware of your breathing, how you contact the floor, and how you are generally. Sense the movement in your chest, in your abdomen, and all around. Ideally, one could learn to sense the movement in each rib relative to the rib above and the rib below. Notice how you sense or picture your ribs, chest, abdomen, back, and sides.

Slowly, roll to either side and sit in your chair.

See if you can breathe freely and continuously as you do that.

Part Four
Step One

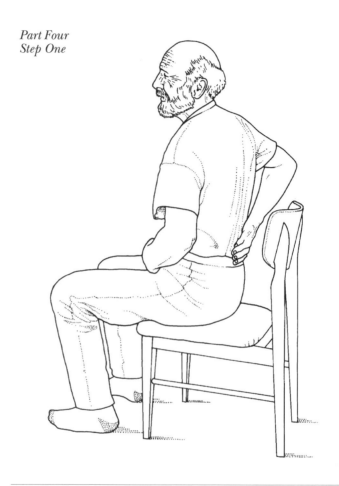

PART FOUR *Sitting*

1 Sit with your feet flat on the floor, without leaning against the back of the chair. Place one hand on your lower abdomen, below the navel, and one hand on your lower back.

Breathe so that your hands move away from each other as you breathe in, and toward each other as you breathe out. You expand forward and backward as you breathe in, your front and your back moving simultaneously. And you contract from the front and back as you breathe out. See if you can do the movement with your breathing only, without tilting your pelvis.

Make this movement as large as comfortable, both expanding and contracting.

Your hands help you sense the movement; they do not push or do anything else. Your pelvis remains in a neutral position, without tilting in either direction.

Do this for several minutes as you sense the movement all around. Move your hands to sense and explore.

Pause and breathe easily for a moment.

2 Now breathe to emphasize the movement in your upper chest and upper back. Expand your upper chest and upper back as you breathe in, and contract front to back as you breathe out. Make this movement as large as you can comfortably.

If you want, use your hands to sense this movement, at least in front. Some people can touch the area between the shoulder blades easily, from above or below, and if that is comfortable for you, you may want to do so.

How clearly can you sense the movement in your back? What are you aware of there, between your shoulder blades? Sense and picture that as clearly as you can.

Any movement of the shoulder blades and upper ribs also involves the collarbones. Can you sense that? The angle between your collarbone and your shoulder blade changes as you breathe. Those two bones meet and articulate in a joint that is essential for the mobility of your arm, although most people have never sensed that.

Briefly rest. Breathe easily.

3 Recall the seesaw movement you did earlier. Take a comfortable amount of air, not too much, and hold your breath for a moment. Squeeze all the muscles in your lower abdomen and lower back to force the air upward. Then squeeze all the muscles in your upper chest and upper back to force the air downward. Again, think of yourself as being like a balloon, partially inflated, with a knot in the end. Push the air upward and downward a few times, then breathe out. Pause as you breathe easily a few times, then repeat this.

Part Four
Step Two

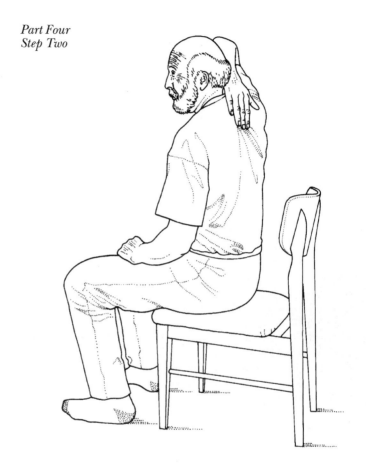

See if you can sense this movement three-dimensionally, in your front, your back, and your sides. Use your hands to help you discover where you move freely and where you can still eliminate any tightness.

Play with making this movement larger or smaller, lighter or faster. Explore different variations, rates, and rhythms. If you like, experiment with doing this movement while breathing lightly. Can you find a way to do that?

Rest for a few moments. Do nothing more. Breathe easily, spontaneously, simply.

4 Begin to expand everywhere, all at once, while you breathe in. Contract all around while you breathe out. Your front and back and sides, above and below.

Start small and gradually make this larger. Do it slowly, so that the movement is complete and comfortable. Use your hands to explore and sense how you are moving everywhere.

Think of your trunk as a balloon. The balloon expands in all directions as it fills with air, and it becomes smaller from all sides as the air is released. Sense the flexibility of that balloon in all directions, your front, sides, back, down into your pelvis and hip joints, up beneath your armpits and shoulders and into your neck.

Yoga practices include many different breathing exercises, called Pranayama, some of which involve elaborate counting and other techniques. While I was a research associate at the Foundation for Mind Research, Bob Masters told me about a yoga teacher he knew and studied with, Swami Karmananda, who had spent many years in India before returning to the United States to write and teach. Swami Karmananda had told Bob about a yogi who was famous for his mastery of Pranayama. Through decades of diligent practice, this great yogi had achieved complete consciousness and mastery over every breath he took. From all around India, other yogis would go to the Himalayas to study with this master.

One day, however, according to Swami Karmananda, this great yogi momentarily forgot about breathing. And he died.

Breathing needs to be spontaneous. The correct way to breathe changes moment by moment, according to where you are and what you are doing.

The best and healthiest way to facilitate better breathing, in my view, is to learn to eliminate acquired or unnecessary inhibitions. Pranayama and other breathing exercises can help you become more aware, yet any technique performed excessively or without awareness can impose new habits on top of existing patterns. Furthermore, any technique may be harmful for some people or at certain times.

Health and vitality, Moshe recognized, are best indicated by spontaneity, and trying to exert conscious control over breathing or other essential functions diminishes spontaneity. Consciousness is neither appropriate nor adequate for controlling breathing. With awareness, you can eliminate any excess tensions or inhibitions and discover more spontaneous ways of acting. Your breathing will improve, and your consciousness will be liberated from an inappropriate burden.

Picture your spine, your head, and your pelvis. Think about your ribs, how they attach to the spine and curve around to your breastbone. Your ribs lift and open as you breathe in, then move downward and inward as you breathe out.

Use your hands if you like to touch and explore, to learn all you can about moving everywhere, even under your armpits.

You might think that this is, possibly, the best way to breathe. In fact, the wisest and most skillful individuals do breathe this way, with no excess strain or effort. You can see that the next time you watch a baby. You also breathed this way when you were a baby, before you learned to inhibit your freedom and flexibility.

What do you notice as you breathe this way? How do you feel, physically and emotionally? Are you calm and peaceful? Invigorated and energetic? Perhaps all of these at once?

Every emotional experience involves certain ways of breathing. As you become more aware and learn to breathe more easily, without habitual tensions or inhibitions, your emotional life will become freer and more spontaneous.

5 See if you can continue breathing easily as you lean forward and stand.

Stand for a moment, and sense the movement everywhere within your trunk. Again, if you like, use your hands to sense your chest, sides, back, up around your shoulders, and down into your pelvis.

And walk.

Observe how you breathe as you walk. Can you continue breathing this fully?

Effortless Sitting

While reading, most people sit in some habitual posture. Are you leaning against the back of a chair or some other support? Are you straight or twisted toward one side? Do you have your feet up on something or your legs crossed? Where are your arms relative to your trunk? Most important of all—are you comfortable?

Young children sit without any back support, arms free, heads erect, looking around and smiling, for as long as they choose. Perhaps you will notice that the next time you see a baby or young child sitting on the floor, a chair, or in a firm stroller. In contrast, most adults lean against something when sitting and fatigue after a few minutes of trying to sit without some support. When you were a baby, you also sat effortlessly without leaning against anything. Somehow you learned your habitual ways of sitting, whatever they may be today.

Babies and young children sit by resting securely on the sitting bones at the base of the pelvis, which is the center and heaviest area of the body and the attachment for the largest and strongest muscles. In this position, the pelvis can move freely, the weight of the head and trunk is supported by the skeleton, and muscles everywhere remain relatively relaxed. For babies, at least, this is the most comfortable, effortless way to sit, which is why they spontaneously choose it. Babies do not have the strength to move inefficiently.

However you choose to sit, this lesson will help you be more aware, skillful, and comfortable.

PART ONE   *Lying on the Floor*

1   Lie on your back with your arms at your sides. Sense how you are right now. Notice how you contact the floor, especially around your pelvis and hip joints. Most of us have only a vague image of the shape of the pelvis, the places where the legs attach at the hip joints, and the sacrum, which is where the spine joins the pelvic bones. If you do this lesson gently and skillfully, you will have much more awareness of these areas afterward.

Bend your legs to place your feet flat on the floor.

Begin to rock your pelvis forward and back. Your lower back lifts from the floor slightly to create a space, then presses the floor and eliminates that space. Do that simply, so your pelvis tilts while remaining in contact with the floor. Lifting your pelvis off the floor involves excessive effort.

You can do most of the work with your legs, pushing and pulling with your feet as they grab the floor. Your abdominal muscles can also help. Push your belly forward as you lift your lower back, and pull your belly in as you press your lower back into the floor.

As always, make this movement smoother, easier, simpler each time you do it. Can you find a way to breathe that assists with moving your abdomen and pelvis? Do this movement 10 or 15 or more times.

Sense the movement in your pelvis as clearly as you can. Also be aware of how your spine moves as you tilt your pelvis. Can you detect any movement in your head or shoulders?

Rest for a moment, with your legs bent and feet flat on the floor.

2   Begin to tilt your legs left and right. Sense this movement in your pelvis as clearly as you can. Your pelvis rolls from side to side, so that one buttock presses into the floor while the other lifts off the floor slightly.

Recall this movement from Lesson Two, *Turning and Twisting*. As you discovered then, having your feet too far from your pelvis or

117

Part One
Step One

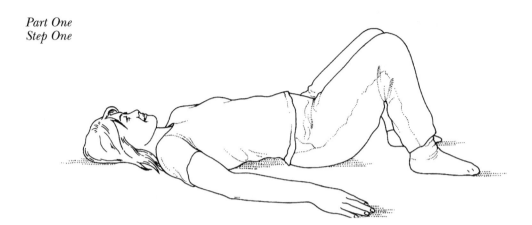

Part One
Step Two

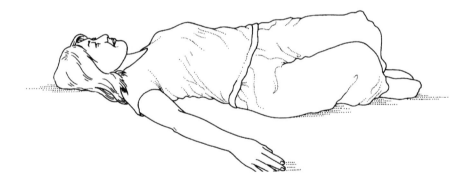

too near restricts the mobility of your pelvis. You also restrict the movement if your feet are too far apart or too close together. Explore various positions for your feet to find where to place them to allow your pelvis to tilt most freely.

Pause, with your knees pointing toward the ceiling and your feet slightly spread.

3 Now tilt your pelvis left and right in the same way while keeping your knees in the middle. Your knees will move a bit forward and back, or up and down, but they do not move left or right.

If that is not clear, again tilt your knees once or twice to sense the movement in your pelvis more clearly. Then continue to move your pelvis without tilting your knees. Begin with a small movement, then make this gradually larger.

Sense what happens in your pelvis and hip joints. And notice how this movement is transmitted along your spine. Where in your back can you sense this rotation?

4 Rest. Extend your legs and lie still. Sense how you contact the floor now.

Imagine a clock on the floor under your pelvis. The dial faces upward, with the 12 toward your head and the 6 toward your feet. That places the 3 to your left and the 9 to your right.

5 Once again, bend your legs so your feet are flat on the floor. Begin to tilt your pelvis forward and back again, to press your lower back into the floor and then lift your lower back off the floor.

When your lower back presses the floor, your weight is toward the 12 on the clock dial. When you lift your lower back, your weight shifts onto your tailbone, which is the 6 on that dial.

If the time were exactly 6:00, you would be shifting your weight along the hands of that clock. Imagine the hands of the clock along the line between your buttocks as you move your pelvis from 12 to 6.

Do this movement a number of times. The image of the dial can help you more accurately sense what you do as you tilt your pelvis forward and back.

Pause briefly.

6 Tilt your pelvis left and right once again, without tilting your legs.

With the image of the dial, this means shifting your weight onto the 3 and the 9. If the time were 9:15 or 3:45, you would be moving your pelvis along the hands of the clock. Again, use the image of the dial to keep the movement even and simple.

Rest. Keep your legs bent or extend them, as you choose.

7 Bend your legs so that the soles of your feet are touching one another. This means that the outsides of the feet are on the floor and your knees point away from each other.

Once again, tilt your pelvis left and right, as you were doing a moment ago.

Notice if this change in the position of your legs affects the range or quality of the movement. What happens in your hip joints now?

Pause again, keeping your legs bent with the soles of your feet touching and your knees apart.

8 Tilt your pelvis forward and back, lifting your lower back slightly and then pressing your lower back into the floor.

Does this position of your legs alter the movement forward and back? Do you sense your hip joints differently, their location and structure?

9 Rest. Extend your legs. Sense how you contact the floor now. Picture your pelvis and legs, and the hip joints where they meet. Is your image of this area more complete than before?

For most people, the pelvis and hip joints are very poorly defined. The actual joints are higher and deeper in the pelvis than most people realize, and closer together. The place that most people identify as the hip joint is a protrusion on the outside of the thigh bone called the greater trochanter. The actual joint is a ball on the head of the thigh bone that rotates within a socket formed in the pelvis. The movements you are doing involve moving your pelvis and that socket, while keeping the ball and thigh bone relatively stable.

Continue to rest as you sense your legs, pelvis, and spine, and your contact with the floor everywhere.

10 Again, bend your legs so that the soles of your feet are touching with your knees apart.

Part One
Step Seven

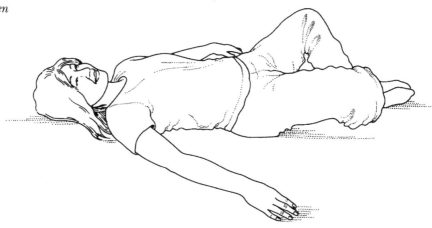

Picture the dial under your pelvis once more, with the 12 and 6 and the 3 and 9 marked. The movements you have been doing involved shifting your weight through the center of the dial. You can also move around the circumference.

Do that. Move your pelvis to the 12. Then shift your weight to 1, 2, 3, 4, 5, 6, 7, 8, 9, 10, 11, and back to 12. Do not try to do this perfectly, or even nicely. Just begin to explore. Start slowly, and use the image of the dial to see if you are finding the 4, skipping the 7, or twisting past the 10. Gradually make this movement smoother and more uniform.

Pause to reorient yourself occasionally, especially if the dial seems twisted or distorted. You might again move forward and back, to 6 and 12, and side to side, to 3 and 9, to redefine those positions. Then resume the movement around the dial. If you still feel that the dial might have been drawn by Salvador Dali, fine—you are learning.

11 Pause. Reverse the direction. Circle the dial counterclockwise. As always, see that you breathe freely.

Make this movement as pleasant, as skillful, as easy, as you can.

Be attentive to any changes in the size or quality of the movement when going in the opposite direction. Is the dial still round?

As you become more aware and able to make slow, simple, circular movements, begin to play with different rates of moving around that dial. Do this faster, or even slower.

12 Do 2 or 3 movements around the dial clockwise, then reverse the direction and do 2 or 3 movements counterclockwise. Continue with that, reversing the direction after every few revolutions.

Sense your chest, your mid-back, your sides, your shoulders, your neck, your head. Notice where you are moving and how this movement in your pelvis involves all of you.

Be attentive to how you are breathing as you move around the dial. Can you breathe freely throughout the movement, or do you hold your breath and tighten at certain places on the dial?

Play with this. Do it faster, slower, larger, smaller. Discover all you can about this movement. Let your comfort be the only constraint: as long as you are comfortable, have fun.

13 Rest. Extend your legs and lie comfortably. Sense how you contact the floor now. Do you picture yourself differently in any way? Be aware of any differences between how you are now and how you were when you began this lesson.

PART TWO *Your Pelvis and Head*

1 Bend your legs so that the soles of your feet are touching, with your knees apart.

Slowly tilt your pelvis forward and back again.

Follow the movement from your pelvis upward, along your spine. What happens in your lower back, mid-back, upper back, neck, and head? Notice how the movement in your pelvis, at one end of your spine, affects your head, at the other end of your spine. Do not do anything to move your head deliberately. Let your head move passively, from the activity in your pelvis.

At what point in the movement of your pelvis does your chin lift toward the ceiling, when your pelvis moves toward 12 or toward 6? At what point does your chin move toward your chest?

Pause.

2 Tilt your pelvis left and right. Sense how this movement is transmitted through your spine. How does your head move now?

Rest for a moment.

3 Move your pelvis around the dial again. Do this a few times in one direction and a few times in the opposite direction.

Sense your lower back, your ribs, chest, and mid-back, the spine between your shoulders, your neck, and your head. See if you can move more freely everywhere, without forcing or trying to achieve anything.

What do you notice about the movement in your head now? Is it free, easy, comfortable?

Rest. Extend your legs.

4 Now imagine a dial underneath your head, similar to the one under your pelvis, but smaller. The numbers are oriented in the same direction. Picture those two dials.

Remember, resting is important for learning. Lie easily for a few moments, breathing freely and evenly.

5 Bend your legs so the soles of your feet are touching again. A few times, move your pelvis to 12 and 6 on its dial while you move your head in the same direction, to 12 and 6 on its dial. The back of your pelvis and the back of your head both tilt to shift the point where each presses the floor.

Sense how your head and pelvis move together in an integrated, connected act. See if you can eliminate any interference in your ribs, chest, and back, so that everywhere participates harmoniously.

Pause for a moment.

6 Move your pelvis to 3 and 9 on its dial while you move your head in the same direction, to 3 and 9 on its dial.

Again, sense the connection between your head and pelvis. Do what you can to make the movement at both ends of your spine smoother, and more coordinated. Notice how your head rolls from left to right on the floor.

Once more, rest for a few moments. Straighten your legs and lie comfortably.

7 Bend your legs again, so that the soles of your feet are touching. You can probably anticipate the next movement.

Picture the two dials, under your pelvis and your head. Slowly begin to move your pelvis around the circumference of its dial while you move your head around its dial. Both go from 1 to 2 to 3 to 4, and on, around the dial.

See if you can make this one, fluid, continuous movement, involving both ends of your spine. Your head and your pelvis are at the same point on their respective dials throughout the movement.

Do this many times, making each movement with less effort.

8 Pause and reverse the direction in your pelvis and in your head. Move your head and your pelvis counterclockwise around their respective dials. Breathe freely.

Again, sense the movement everywhere, with as much detail as you can. Use the image of the dials on the floor to make the movement smoother and more uniform. If you become confused or disoriented at any point, pause, picture the dials, and then resume the movement.

Be aware of your whole head, your mouth, nose and eyes, your chin and ears, the top of your head. Does your nose make a circle in the air? What about your chin, can you also picture a circle there? Or is that an ellipse? Or an egg shape? What kind of shape do your ears make in space?

9 Do 3 or 4 movements in one direction, then reverse and do 3 or 4 movements in the opposite direction.

Continue to reverse the direction after every few circles. Can you reverse the direction in your head and pelvis in a way that is truly simultaneous?

Notice where you choose to reverse the direction. Do you always reverse at the 12 or the 6? See if you can reverse the circles at various points in the movement. Play with reversing the direction in different ways.

Also play with varying the speed of moving around the dials. As long as you breathe freely and make this easy, explore as many variations of circling and changing direction as you can. Have fun and learn.

10 Rest. Extend your legs. Lie still. Compare how you are now, your contact with the floor and your overall awareness, with how you were at the beginning of this lesson.

As I have mentioned, the largest and strongest muscles you have are those that cross your hip joints and attach your pelvis and legs. These muscles provide the power for everything you do. The head contains all the teleceptors, the sensory receptors for distant information—eyes, ears, and nose. Skillful movement requires good coordination between head and pelvis. Your head orients you to the world and selects the direction of any movement, while your pelvis provides the power for movement.

You might want to play with these movements in bed, before you go to sleep or in the morning when you wake. Or you can lie on the floor, for the clearer feedback of a firmer surface. You can do these movements with your legs in different positions, even asymmetrical positions. The movement can be small or large, fast or slow. As long as you move in ways that are pleasant and interesting, you will continue to learn and improve.

11 Bend your legs so your feet are flat on the floor. Tilt your pelvis forward and backward, simply.

Forget about the dials. Let your head move passively. Just tilt your pelvis to press your lower back against the floor and lift your lower back off the floor.

Compare this movement now with before. How far does your pelvis tilt? How easily? How do you sense your legs and hip joints? What are you doing with your abdominal muscles? Are they helping? Sense how this movement is transmitted through your spine to your head.

Part Two
Step Eleven

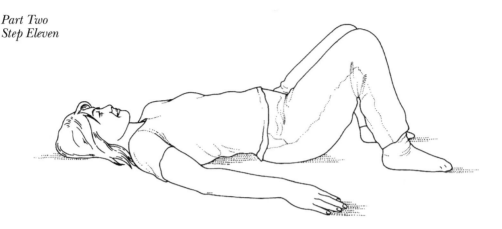

Notice how you are breathing. Are you spontaneously coordinating your breathing with the movement in some way?

Rest briefly.

12 Think about rolling to your side to stand. First, however, sense your pelvis and picture how you can begin rolling to your side there, from your center. Since that area contains the largest and strongest muscles, you want to roll and stand in a way that does the work there, efficiently, with no excess effort elsewhere.

After you think that through for a few moments, slowly, smoothly roll to either side and sit in your chair.

PART THREE *Sitting*

1 Sit forward on your chair, not leaning against the back, with your feet flat on the floor.

Tilt your pelvis forward and backward, to rock on your sitting bones. As always, be attentive to breathing easily.

Sense your pelvis moving relative to your legs, the bending in your hip joints. Let your spine remain relatively straight and long as you tilt your pelvis forward and back. Notice how far your head and shoulders move.

Pause.

126

Part Three
Step One

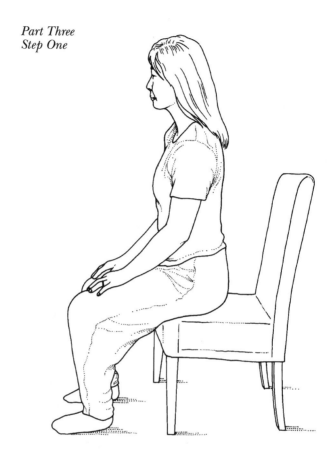

2 Tilt your pelvis forward and backward, but now let your whole spine curve like a **C**, first in one direction, then in the opposite direction.

See if you can do this smoothly, simply, so that the **C** curve is continuous from top to bottom. Reduce the movement in your head and neck so that they flow with the pelvis. If you were observing yourself from the side, you would see that moving the head too far breaks the curve. If the **C** curve is even, your head stays almost directly above your pelvis.

127

Part Three
Step Two

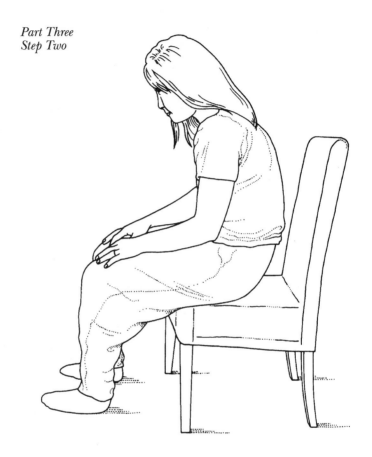

Do this movement many times.

Make this movement as smooth and easy, continuous and comfortable as you can.

Recall what you learned in Lesson One, *Bending and Breathing*, about how you can coordinate your breathing with the movement to make it easier. Also recall Lesson Four, *Uninhibited Breathing*, and see if you can eliminate any inhibitions in your breathing to improve the range and quality of this movement.

3 Rest. Simply sit without leaning against the back of your chair.

Part Three
Step Two

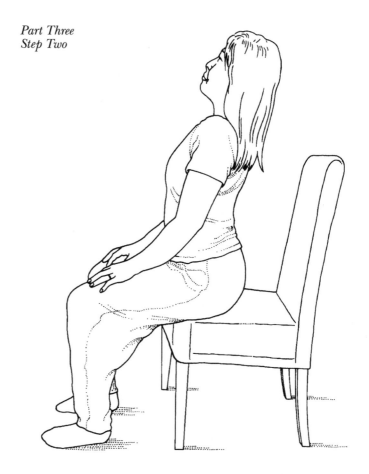

Sense how you are sitting, especially the contact of your sitting bones on the chair.

Imagine that you are now sitting on a clock dial. Picture that dial oriented in the same way relative to your pelvis as when you were lying on the floor. This means that the 6 is toward your front with the 12 in back. The 3 is again on your left and the 9 on your right.

4   Begin to tilt your pelvis forward and backward again, letting your spine curve like a C. When you tilt your pelvis forward and arch

your back, you shift your weight onto the 6. When you tilt your pelvis backward and round your spine, you shift your weight onto the 12.

Sense the movement from the base of your pelvis to the top of your head. Your whole spine arches and rounds. Observe your legs, hip joints, pelvis, lower back, mid-back, ribs and sides, chest, shoulder blades, neck, and head.

Pause and rest.

5 Now tilt your pelvis left and right, shifting your weight onto the 3 and the 9 on this dial. When you lift the right sitting bone and shift your weight to the left, you are on 3. When you shift your weight right by lifting the left sitting bone, you are on the 9.

Recall the movements from Lesson Three, *Leaning and Lifting,* and do this in the way that curves your spine like a C, first in one direction, then in the opposite direction, the mirror image of that C. Your ribs squeeze together on one side and fan apart on the opposite side. Your head can again remain directly over your pelvis.

Make this movement as large as you can.

Sense the movement all through your spine, your ribs, chest, and back. Do whatever you can to make this movement freer, easier, larger.

Rest for a few moments.

6 Begin to move your pelvis to shift your weight around the circumference of the clock dial. Move onto each number in succession.

Start slowly and breathe easily.

If you feel confused or lost, slow down. Or stop and reorient yourself to the dial by simply doing the movement forward and back, then left and right.

See if you can move smoothly through each point on the dial, without skipping any numbers or distorting the circle in any way. Is the dial really round and uniform? Or is it a bit oval, or egg-shaped?

Pause.

Part Three
Step Five

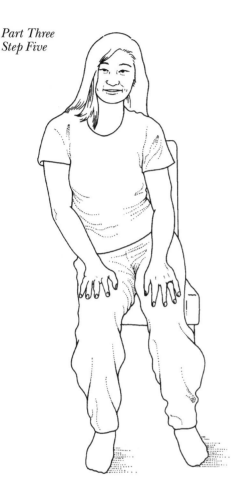
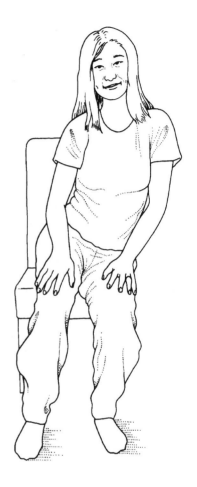

7 Reverse the direction. Continue to circle your pelvis around the dial, going the opposite way.

Gradually make the movement larger. Remember the dial and use that image to keep it really round and fluid. How large a movement can you make? Is it a small desk clock, or can you do the movement as if going around a large wall clock? See how large you can make the movement, as long as you maintain the quality of the movement.

131

8 Do 2 or 3 movements in one direction, pause, reverse that, and do 2 or 3 movements in the opposite direction.

When you paused and reversed direction, where were you on the dial? Were you at the 12 or 6? Play with reversing the direction at different points.

As you continue to do that, sense your sitting bones on the chair. Also sense your chest, your back, your ribs, your shoulders. Are you aware of your head moving in space? What is happening in your shoulder blades? What about your breastbone or sternum— can you picture the movement there?

9 Rest. Sit easily and do nothing. Simply be aware of how you are sitting now.

Notice the position of your pelvis and your head. Sense the amount of effort you use to sit. Be aware of your breathing, the range and quality of movement in your abdomen and chest, in your ribs all around.

For a few moments, lean against the back of your chair and sit in some more familiar way.

While leaning back, sense the position of your pelvis and how your sitting bones contact the chair. Does sitting this way alter how you breathe? Simply compare and contrast these two ways of sitting.

PART FOUR *Sitting: Pelvis and Head*

1 Sit without leaning against the back of your chair, with your feet flat on the floor.

Again, tilt your pelvis from 6 to 12 on the imaginary dial a few times, with your spine curving like a C.

Notice the position of your head when your pelvis is at 6 and at 12, both relative to your pelvis and relative to the room around you.

2 Now do the movement from 3 to 9, curving your spine like a C.

When your pelvis is at 3 and at 9, observe where your head is, again relative to your pelvis and relative to the room.

3 Move your pelvis around the circumference of the dial. Do this slowly, and be attentive to the position of your head throughout the movement.

When your pelvis is at 12, 6, 3, or 9, your head can be in the same position relative to your pelvis as when you were only moving forward and back or left and right. Is it?

4 Reverse the direction after every few rotations. Make the movement as large as comfortable, slowly, easily. Sense your head moving in space as you make circles with your pelvis.

What kind of movement is your head making? Is it a circle? Can you picture that clearly?

Do what you can to make the movement of your head more even and simple.

5 Gradually make the movement smaller. Let the dial become smaller each time you go around, until it is no more than a small watch. Do a few movements in one direction and a few movements in the opposite direction.

See if you can make that movement so small that someone observing you would not detect any activity. Continue to move your pelvis around the dial, but invisibly.

Sense what you are doing everywhere, your pelvis and head, your spine and ribs all around.

6 Rest for a few moments. Do you need to lean against the back of the chair, or can you rest without leaning? If you want to lean, do so. Let that be a choice, not just a habit.

7 Once more, sit without leaning against the back of your chair.

Tilt your pelvis left and right, so that your spine curves like a C toward each side. Breathe freely with that movement.

How does this compare with when you did it before? Is it easier? Are you more aware? Notice what you are doing in your ribs all

133

around, your spine, your chest and back, your shoulders and head.

Gradually make the movement smaller until it would be undetectable to someone watching you. See if you can find the place where you are completely balanced left and right, so the muscles on each side are equally at ease, even as you continue to do the smallest movement you can.

8 Beginning from that balanced position, tilt your pelvis forward and back, with your spine curving like a C.

Compare this movement with before. Sense the range and the quality. What do you notice now? Can you sense movement in your ribs all around, your spine, chest, back, shoulders, and head?

Gradually make this movement smaller until it becomes imperceptible. See if you can discover where you are completely balanced forward and back, the muscles in front and in back equally relaxed, and the weight of your head supported completely by the spine, so that sitting is totally effortless.

9 Pause, poised and balanced on your sitting bones. Rest that way.

Think about what sitting this way involves. When you are balanced like this, you could tilt your pelvis in any direction with equal ease, instantaneously, without any preparation or effort.

How do you feel while sitting this way? Are you comfortable?

The word *comfortable* is actually French and literally means *with strength,* which suggests that we are most comfortable when we are strong and secure, able to act effectively. That is quite different from the common notion of being comfortable when collapsed into an overstuffed chair or sofa.

10 Stand. Sense the relative position of your head, your pelvis, and your feet.

How is your weight supported? Do you sense your skeleton more completely than usual, so that you stand in a way that is easy and light?

And walk.

Notice how you step, and how you shift your weight from one step to the next. What are you aware of in the way you walk? How does this compare with your normal way of walking? Do you like this feeling, this way of walking?

PART FIVE *From Sitting to Standing*

1 Return to your chair and sit. Now stand again. And sit once more.

Notice how you do that. What do you do to move from sitting to standing and back? How do you move your head, your arms, your pelvis? How much effort is required, and which muscles do the work?

Observe what you do with your head and shoulders. And see if you do anything with your feet. Do you need to prepare to stand by sliding your feet closer under you?

2 Sit as you were a moment ago, balanced and effortless, with your feet flat on the floor.

Keep your spine more or less straight, and begin to rock forward on your sitting bones and back to the neutral, balanced position. The only movement is at your hip joints, where your pelvis and legs meet. The work is all done by those powerful muscles that cross your hip joints.

Rock gently forward and to neutral. Be sure you breathe easily as you do that.

3 Gradually make the forward movement larger, so that your shoulders move further over your knees each time you rock forward. Leave your arms at your sides and allow them to swing easily. If you rest your hands on your thighs the movement of your shoulders and upper back will be inhibited.

Notice what you are doing with your head and eyes. If you are rocking simply, moving only at the hip joints and keeping your spine more or less straight, as you rock forward your head moves in an arc downward, and your eyes look toward the floor. Your eyes look forward again as you rock back to the neutral position.

135

Part Five
Step Three

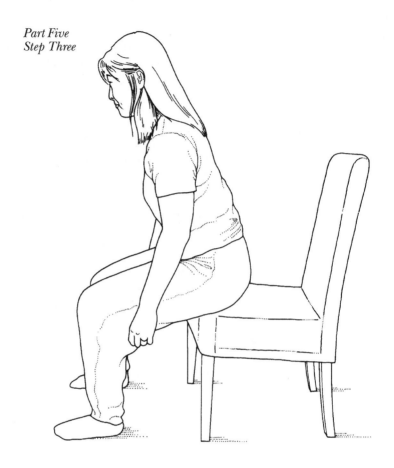

See if you can rock in this way very smoothly and simply. Again, as always, the best indicator of aware and skillful movement is easy continuous breathing. Any tightening in your chest or inhibiting of your breathing indicates unnecessary effort.

Rest. Simply think about this movement for a moment. What would you need to do to make this movement larger? Can you move more freely than you have been at your hip joints?

4 Rock forward and back to neutral again. Continue doing that, easily.

Part Five
Step Four

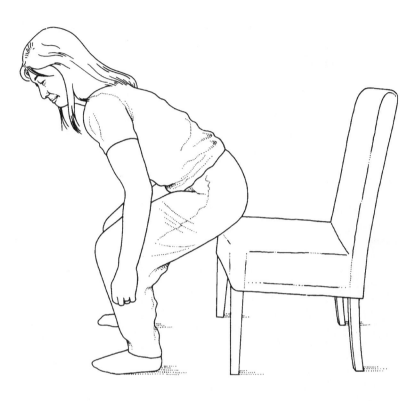

As you rock forward each time, notice how you shift your weight. As your shoulders move toward your knees, you begin to shift more weight onto your feet. If the forward movement is large, you will sense more weight on your feet than on your pelvis.

The next time your weight is over your feet, see if you can begin to lift your pelvis a bit off the chair. Do this only if it is easy. Then lower your pelvis and lean back again to sit straight. Be sure you lean your pelvis far enough forward to sense your weight clearly over your feet before you do anything to lift your pelvis. And only lift your pelvis an inch or two, for just a moment.

Be aware of your knees and feet. In order to lift yourself easily, they need to be aligned to support your weight. If either your knees or your feet are twisted outward or inward, lifting your pelvis will be more difficult.

After the second summer of the Amherst Feldenkrais training program, in 1981, Moshe asked me to accompany him to Florida where he was to be interviewed for a series of cable television programs.

We arrived at the studio the first morning and saw a typical talk show set: a sofa and coffee table, an easy chair, and, in the background, a bookcase filled with Reader's Digest Condensed Books, probably from a garage sale. The director asked Moshe to sit in the chair, and said that the medical doctor who hosted the show would sit at one end of the sofa, near Moshe.

Moshe sat on that large cushioned chair as if it were a stool, well forward from the back. After a few minutes the director asked Moshe to please lean back and sit normally so they could adjust the lights. Moshe told the director that he was most comfortable sitting forward and would do so throughout the programs.

The crew worked on the lighting for almost an hour. Then the director again approached Moshe, "Would you mind leaning back? Sitting forward casts a shadow on the back of the chair and it looks terrible on the monitors." Moshe repeated that he preferred to sit as he was.

After the crew tried adjusting the lights for another 40 minutes or so, the director came over to where I was standing. "Could you explain to him about the trouble we are having with the lights and why it would be better if he sat back on the chair?" I knew better and refused to try. "That's how he's going to sit. You'll just have to work with it." They played with the lights for another half hour before beginning to tape the first show.

They taped two or three half-hour programs that day, and taping continued the following day. Throughout, Moshe sat on that easy chair as if on a stool. The doctor sat leaning against the back of the sofa most of the time, slightly twisted, usually with one leg crossed over the other, occasionally putting his feet up on the coffee table.

Most of us sit something like the doctor, especially on sofas or easy chairs, leaning back, crossing our legs, putting our feet up. Moshe occasionally did these things, but never for more than a few moments. His way of sitting or changing position, it seemed to me, was the opposite of the doctor and most people. Most of us occasionally sit up, but only briefly, when preparing to stand or while shifting from one position to another.

In the afternoon of the second day of filming, the doctor began a new segment by asking about sitting. Moshe explained that he sat without any back support because that was how he was most comfortable. Then Moshe demonstrated that his balanced, effortless way of sitting allowed him to move freely in any direction, forward, back, left, right, up, or down, without any hesitation or preliminary preparation.

Moshe then turned to the doctor and pointed his finger. "Look how you're sitting. If there were a fire or other emergency and you had to stand instantly, you'd be killed. Your chest is collapsed, your breathing is impaired, and your back is strained. Someone who always sits like that will end up with back pain and other difficulties." The doctor blushed and admitted that he had suffered from chronic back pain for many years.

Almost a year passed before I actually saw the video. I was not surprised to find this last exchange edited out.

Breathe freely. Can you find a way to breathe that enables you to rock forward and lift your pelvis more easily?

Rest for a few moments. Sit comfortably and do nothing. This movement, if unfamiliar, involves more effort than you might realize.

5 Begin to lean forward and rock on your sitting bones again. If you can do so easily, let your pelvis lift slightly off the chair.

The next time your pelvis lifts, straighten your legs and stand. Then bend your legs and move your pelvis down toward the chair along the same trajectory until you are sitting again. If you can do so easily, stand and sit this way several times. If you sense any strain, do this movement only in your imagination.

When your leg muscles work efficiently, you can do this very smoothly, without any pushing or straining. Lean forward to shift your weight onto the feet, then straighten your legs to stand. Reverse that to sit again.

6 Sit and rest for a few more moments. Sense your hip joints, sitting bones, and the structure of your pelvis all around.

This way of moving from sitting to standing or standing to sitting can be quite difficult for many people, even for some who are young and athletic. Yet it is not a feat of strength. I have seen many elderly people who never exercise do this beautifully. As you become more aware of your pelvis and hip joints, you will learn to coordinate the muscles there more efficiently. Since those are the largest and strongest muscles in the body, as I have mentioned before, learning to use them skillfully will help you with everything you do.

I encourage you to play with these movements each day for a few minutes. Each of us sits and stands many times every day, so you have many opportunities to explore ways to make this simpler and easier. This is an excellent way to simultaneously lengthen and strengthen all the muscles at the hip joints, especially if you do the movements slowly. You might even pause at various points in the movement and see if you can breathe freely when poised somewhere between sitting and standing.

I want to emphasize that I am not telling you to sit like this or to stand like that. There is nothing wrong with sitting with your legs crossed, or leaning against the back of the chair, or doing whatever you like—as long as you are aware. If you habitually sit in one position or lean against the chair at every opportunity, however, you will find yourself becoming less comfortable when doing anything else.

When you are more aware of your pelvis, your hip joints, and how you balance, you can sit comfortably and move freely wherever you are. You can sit on a simple stool, an overstuffed sofa, or on the floor, all comfortably. If you want, you can play with the movements in this lesson, tilting or circling your pelvis, on any kind of seat, while leaning against something, or even with your legs crossed. You can learn to sit effortlessly at a movie or restaurant, in your car, even while reading or writing or operating a computer. Remember, the benefits come from awareness, not from stretching or strengthening muscles.

Elegant Walking

Walking is difficult for many people, especially the elderly, for whom problems with stairs and curbs are so common that these troubles are sometimes considered inevitable traits of old age. Yet these and related difficulties may be better explained by lack of awareness than by age alone. Except when experiencing pain, we rarely think about how we walk. Do you know how your pelvis moves as you walk? Have you ever thought about that?

In this lesson, you learn to walk more comfortably and efficiently. The awareness and skill you gain can also improve running, dancing, golf, tennis, and many other activities. If you learn to walk more elegantly now, you may be skipping at the age of 90 or 100.

For this lesson, you will need a place to stand where you can rest your hands on something for balance, such as a table, a bookcase, or the back of a tall chair. For the walking and standing movements, a wooden floor will give more reliable feedback than a deep carpet, and bare feet may be preferred to shoes. As in the other lessons, you will also be doing some of the movements while lying down.

This lesson incorporates movements from each of the preceding five. If you have any difficulty, I suggest you review the other lessons, with added attention to how you move your pelvis, and then return to this one.

Remember, the less effort you use, the more quickly you will learn. Repeat each movement many times to sense clearly what you are doing. If you have any history of back problems, rest whenever you want to. You can also pause at any point in the lesson, then resume another time by reviewing to wherever you stopped.

Have fun with this lesson, especially the final part, which is best done playfully.

PART ONE   *Walking and Shifting Weight*

1   Walk around for a few moments. Observe how you walk normally.

Sense what happens in your legs, pelvis, back, head, and arms. Notice how your arms swing, the range and quality of movement and how that relates to your legs. Be aware of how your feet contact the floor. Be attentive also to the mobility in your head and eyes. Some people fixate the head or eyes while sensing and thinking about how they are walking; as you know from the previous lessons, when you stiffen anywhere, you distort the way you move everywhere. A useful way to observe yourself, remember, is to shift your attention from moment to moment, from one area to the overall picture of yourself then to another area.

When thinking about walking, people typically focus on the leg that is stepping forward. Were you doing that? Can you be more aware of the supporting leg? What else might you notice?

Pause for a moment. Stand where you can rest your hands comfortably on something. Even if you do not need to rest your hands on something for balance, please do so. The more secure you are, the easier it is for you to be aware and learn.

2   Simply think of stepping forward with your right foot. Do that a number of times: think about stepping forward, then about returning to neutral standing. Notice what you do as you prepare to step. Where do you sense the first impulse for the movement? Do you begin with your foot, your knee, or somewhere else?

Now actually step forward with your right foot, then return your foot to where it was. Do this slowly, attentively, several times. You can do it while lifting your foot a few inches only, or even less.

How do you initiate the movement of stepping? Where do you move first? What do you do before you lift your foot?

Sense how the first movement occurs in your pelvis and hip joints. That may seem obvious after your experience with the previous lessons, yet it is a surprise to most people. Before you can step with your right foot, you have to shift your weight onto your left leg, which necessarily involves moving your pelvis in some way. You cannot lift your leg while it is supporting you, at least not without falling.

3 Shift your weight onto your right leg then onto your left leg. Do not walk. Do not even lift either foot. Simply shift your weight onto one leg and then onto the other. Shift your weight fully, so that each leg alternately becomes completely free.

Sense how you do that. See what you can discover about how you move your pelvis, hip joints, and back as you shift your weight from one leg to the other. Do this movement many times.

Breathe freely and keep your eyes and head free. One way to be sure your head is free is to look around as you do this movement, or at least think about looking around.

To walk elegantly, you need to begin to be more aware of your supporting leg. When you shift your weight completely onto one leg, you can then step effortlessly with the other. With a secure supporting leg, you can take a large or small step, up a stair or down from a curb.

4 Walk again, slowly. Sense how you move your pelvis to stand on your right leg or on your left leg.

What do you notice? Does your pelvis move from side to side in a straight line? Does it twist? Or tilt? Is the movement symmetrical?

Walk, and be especially attentive to the leg you stand on during each step. Be sure your head and eyes are free. Let your arms swing easily. Walk as freely as you can while remaining aware of your pelvis and hip joints.

Part Two *Lying on Your Back*

1   Lie on your back, with your legs extended and your arms at your sides.

Rest briefly.

Sense how you contact the floor. Observe especially the contact your legs and pelvis make with the floor. Notice if either side seems longer, heavier, more present.

2   Slide the right side of your pelvis along the floor toward your right shoulder. This makes your right leg, and your whole right side, shorter. Then lengthen again. Move from your pelvis to shorten and lengthen your right side, without lifting or bending your right knee.

Sense the movement throughout your right side, along your spine, and in your ribs all around.

Pause for a moment.

3   Now slide the left side of your pelvis along the floor to make that side shorter. Shorten and lengthen your left side.

Compare the movement on your left with the movement on your right. Are there any differences in how far, or how easily, you move? What happens on your right side as you shorten and lengthen on the left?

People with back problems sometimes believe their pain is caused by one leg being shorter than the other, and I have met many people who were told this by chiropractors. That may be true for a few people, but in most cases when one leg seems shorter the person is unaware and tensing muscles on one side, either in the lower back or around the hip joint. In my experience, when someone is aware and knows how to move freely, one leg can be slightly shorter without difficulties. A short leg seems to be a problem only if the difference is significant, as sometimes occurs if the leg was broken at some time or operated on.

4   Alternately shorten your right side and then shorten your left side. See if you can do this without any lifting, either in the hip joint or in the knee. Simply slide your legs along the floor.

Part Two
Step Two

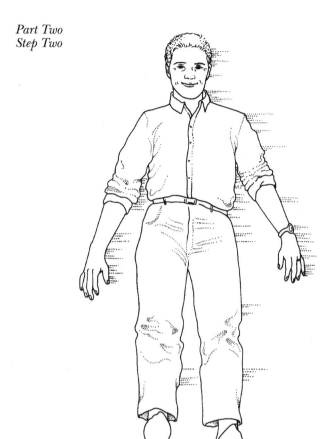

The movement comes from the pelvis and involves all of yourself. When one side shortens, the other side has to lengthen, of course. For now, let your attention be on whichever side is becoming shorter and let any lengthening occur more or less passively.

Sense what you do in your ribs and throughout your trunk, especially on whichever side is becoming shorter.

5 Rest for a moment. Sense how you are now, your contact with the floor and general awareness.

Roll slowly to one side and stand.

PART THREE *A Second Way of Walking*

1 Again, stand and rest your hands on something for balance.

Move the right side of your pelvis up toward the right shoulder until your right foot leaves the floor, then lengthen your right side again to stand normally. You shorten the right side in the same way you did while lying on the floor. See if you can do this so your pelvis moves straight up and down, simply. Each time you lower your right leg, let your weight shift to a balanced standing position.

Notice how this movement involves your whole right side, from your pelvis to your shoulder and neck. Breathe easily.

Pause.

2 Lift the left side of your pelvis. Your left foot leaves the floor and you shift your weight onto your right leg. Then lower your left side and stand normally.

As you shorten your left side and return to balanced standing, sense what happens in your chest, ribs, and back, on both sides.

Again, pause briefly.

3 Lift your legs alternately by shortening one side and then the other. See if you can do that so your pelvis on the side you are lifting moves straight up and down.

Compare the movement on the left with the movement on the right. Does one side lift more easily? Sense how you move in your pelvis, your hip joints, and all through your trunk.

Continue this movement, more slowly. You shorten one side and lift that foot, return to balanced standing, then shorten the other side and lift the other foot.

Sense the movement of transition from one leg to the other. Notice how you move your pelvis as you shift.

Part Three
Step One

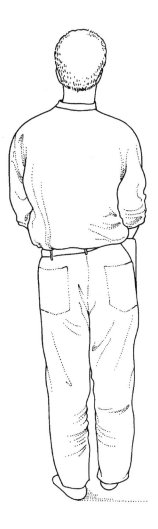

Also be aware of the leg that is supporting you. Does your supporting leg bend or straighten as you lift and lower the other leg? When your weight is all on one leg, is that knee bent, comfortably straight, or locked? Remember, the more securely you stand on one leg, the more skillfully you can lift the other.

Rest. Stand with your weight on both legs, evenly.

147

4 As you stand, think about what you have been doing. When either foot is lifted in this way, from the pelvis, can you move the foot forward a bit before lowering it?

Turn away from whatever you are resting your hands on and begin to do that. Lift one side of your pelvis, move the raised foot forward slightly, then lower that foot and side of your pelvis. Alternate that movement on your right and left sides. Take a number of small steps in this way.

Sense the movement all through your trunk. Continue to be especially attentive to how you shift your weight and to how securely you stand on your supporting leg during each step.

As you do this, rest your hands on the large bones that mark the top of your pelvis on either side. Your hands can help you sense the lifting in the right side of your pelvis as you move that leg forward, and the lifting in the left side of your pelvis as you move that leg forward.

5 This way of walking may seem stiff and zombie-like, yet that is only because you are doing it so deliberately. See if you can make the movement more fluid and natural. Play with this way of walking.

Sense the movement everywhere as you do that. Breathe freely, to allow your ribs and trunk to move easily.

This may still seem awkward, yet some people normally move the pelvis this way as they walk. Now that you are becoming aware, you may find that you observe more accurately how other people move.

Walk for a few more moments, while lifting one side of your pelvis to raise the corresponding foot. Make this simpler and easier. Let your arms swing freely, your knees bend slightly, and your head and eyes turn to look around. You might even be able to smile at the same time.

PART FOUR   *Lying on Your Back*

1 Lie on your back on the floor and rest. Do nothing for a moment.

After childhood, Moshe believed, all learning involves things you already know how to do, but learning a new way to do them. He insisted that you can only do something well when you have at least three choices about how to do it. You now know two ways of shifting your weight while walking: your habitual way, which for most people involves moving the pelvis more or less in a straight line from one side to the other; and this new way, lifting one side of the pelvis.

Can you think of a third possibility? How else can you move your pelvis?

2 Push the right side of your pelvis in the direction of your right foot. Then release that push. Do that a number of times, sliding the right side of your pelvis in the direction of your right foot, downward.

Pushing from the pelvis in this way lengthens your right leg on the floor. You might imagine that there is something on the floor beneath your heel and you want to push it away from you. See if you can do that without lifting or bending or otherwise working in your right knee, ankle, or foot. Your right leg simply slides along the floor, downward and back to neutral.

3 Do the same movement on your left side. Lengthen your left side by moving your pelvis in the direction of your left foot. Make your left leg longer, then release that, a number of times.

Sense that movement in your ribs, your chest, your back, all through your left side.

4 Lengthen your legs alternately. Be attentive mostly to the side that is lengthening. Of course, the other side becomes shorter at the same time, which means that this is similar to the previous movement. The main difference is in your attention and emphasis, now on the side that is lengthening. Again, keep the movement simple and easy, without lifting, bending, or twisting either leg.

Part Four
Step Two

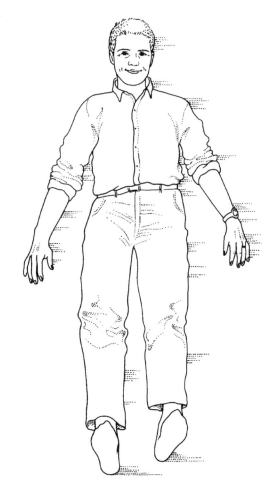

Sense how this movement involves your pelvis, back, ribs, and sides. Are there areas that seem unclear or immobile? Can you sense any movement between your shoulder blades, in your mid-back and upper back?

5 Rest for a moment. Breathe easily. Sense how you contact the floor.

Roll slowly to either side and stand.

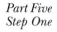

Part Five
Step One

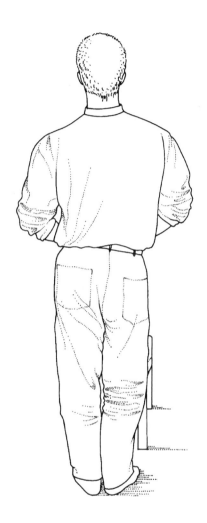

PART FIVE *A Third Way of Walking*

1 Again, stand where you can rest your hands on something for balance.

Shift your weight onto the left leg as you move the right side of your pelvis downward, toward the floor, bending your right knee to make room for that downward movement. Your left leg remains straight, without locking your knee, to support your weight securely.

Then return to balanced standing. Do this a number of times. See if you can make this movement simple and easy.

Sense how your pelvis tilts to shift all your weight onto your left leg as you lower your right hip joint toward the floor. Notice the movement in your back, your ribs, your chest.

2 Now do the same thing to the other side a few times. Shift your weight onto your right leg while you lower the left side of your pelvis and bend your left leg. Then return to balanced standing. Repeat that a number of times.

Rest for a moment.

3 Alternate those movements. Shift your weight onto the right leg as you lower the left side of your pelvis. Then shift your weight onto your left leg as you lower the right side of your pelvis. Do this slowly, smoothly, simply. Be as attentive to returning to neutral as you are to lowering either side.

Be especially aware of the supporting leg. People with knee problems often tend to lock or wiggle that knee as they shift weight onto or off of the standing leg. Notice how the hip joint, knee, and foot of your standing leg align and relate. Does that knee seem to point inward, toward the big toe and opposite leg, or outward, over your little toe? Can you sense how your weight is supported through the knee and long bones in your leg and in your ankle and heel and foot?

When you stand securely, your weight is supported by the skeleton, not the muscles. If you are not quite secure on your supporting leg, you will tend to hold your breath, stiffen your chest or neck, or fixate your eyes and stare at something. As you learn to stand more securely, you can intentionally move your head and eyes to look around. Sense the ease and mobility throughout your trunk as you stand with your weight on one leg or the other.

In our society, some women exaggerate moving the pelvis, considering it sexy, while many men minimize movements of the pelvis to avoid looking effeminate. Whether you are a man or a woman, you can be aware and allow your pelvis to tilt easily, freely, enjoyably, neither exaggerating nor inhibiting. If you choose to, of course, you can always emphasize or minimize that movement.

4 Continue to shift your weight onto either leg as you lower the opposite side of your pelvis. Each time you shift your weight onto one straight leg, bend the other leg a bit more, at the hip joint, knee, and ankle. See if you can then lift the foot slightly off the floor. Only lift your foot when it becomes easy, when you are standing securely on the supporting leg and bending the free leg adequately.

Remember, the more securely you stand on one leg, the more fully and completely you can release and bend the other leg. See if you can lower one side of your pelvis and smoothly bend that hip joint, knee, and ankle to lift your foot smoothly, effortlessly. Be sure you breathe easily as you do that.

As this movement becomes more secure and familiar, you may want to rest your hands on your pelvis. Sense how your pelvis tilts so that the side on which you are standing is higher, while the other side of your pelvis is lower. If you have your hands on your pelvis, you will be able to sense and eliminate any tightening as you lift your foot.

Sense what happens in your ribs all around on both sides as you tilt your pelvis and shift all of your weight onto either leg. On the side that is free, sense the weight of your leg pulling downward. Breathe easily and see if you can look around as you do this.

Continue to do this movement, being especially aware of the moment when you are shifting your weight from one leg to the other. Sense how your pelvis tilts as you shift your weight. You may want to do this movement more slowly, to sense more clearly and make this transition more smoothly.

Pause for a brief rest at any time if you become tired or inattentive.

5 Now each time you lift one foot, move it forward a bit. Start to walk, slowly, taking very small steps. The idea is not to get anywhere but only to discover a way to walk while tilting your pelvis

153

and shifting your weight in this way. There is nowhere you need to go right now.

Walk this way for a few moments, with your attention on the supporting leg so that your pelvis tilts freely. See if you can make this way of walking more simple and fluid.

Again, if you observe people, you will find some who clearly tilt their pelvises this way with each step.

PART SIX *Lying on Your Back*

1   Lie on the floor and rest for a moment. Sense your pelvis and how you contact the floor everywhere, all along your spine, from your pelvis to your head. Notice the movement in your ribs all around as you breathe.

2   Begin to lengthen one side while you shorten the other. Do this so the movement involves your whole trunk. Notice especially the movement in your ribs all around as you breathe easily.

Sense what happens along your spine from your pelvis and tailbone through to your neck and head. Notice how your ribs squeeze together on one side as they fan apart on the opposite side.

Pause briefly.

3   Bend your legs so your knees are in the air and your feet are flat on the floor. Tilt your knees left and right. Allow your feet to pivot on the floor. Do that many times.

Your pelvis rolls on the floor as you tilt your knees, and that rolling is transmitted along your spine to your head. This rolling in your pelvis and spine also moves your ribs. You are moving your pelvis in a different direction than a moment ago, yet your ribs also fan apart on one side while squeezing together on the other side.

Tilt your knees freely, easily, playfully. Sense the movement in your ribs and all through your trunk as clearly as you can.

Pause and extend your legs.

4 Again, lengthen one side as you shorten the opposite side.

Has the previous movement enabled you to sense and move your ribs and upper back more freely or easily? Compare how your ribs are moving now with how they moved when you were tilting your legs.

Make this movement as large and fluid as you can. Be aware of what happens on both sides and throughout your trunk as you do that.

5 Rest again. Lie still and do nothing. For a few moments, sense how you contact the floor as you breathe easily.

Roll to either side and stand.

PART SEVEN *Standing, One Leg in Front of the Other*

1 Stand where you can rest either hand on something for balance. Take a normal-sized step forward with one leg and stay like that. Stand with one foot in front of the other a comfortable distance.

2 Shift your weight onto the forward leg, and back to the rear leg, completely, a number of times.

Throughout the movement, keep both feet in contact with the floor, at least partially. When you stand securely on the forward leg, the toes of the free rear foot can touch the floor for balance. When you stand securely on the rear leg, you can assist your balance by leaving the heel or toes of the forward foot on the floor.

Sense how you stand when your weight is all on the forward leg or all on the rear leg. The leg you stand on can be straight and secure, without locking the knee. If you sense any tightness or strain, it means you have not shifted your weight fully or efficiently and muscles somewhere are working excessively. The leg that is not supporting you can be completely free, either straight or slightly bent.

Notice how you shift your weight. Sense the movement in your pelvis and throughout your trunk. See if you can shift your weight smoothly, easily, with no excess effort anywhere. The more

155

Part Seven
Step Two

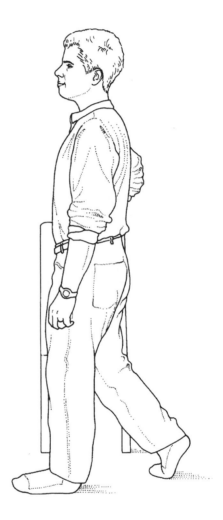

skillfully you move from your pelvis and hip joints, the freer your head and trunk will be.

3 Reverse your legs to stand with the opposite foot in front, with your feet a comfortable distance apart, as if you have just taken a normal step. A number of times, shift your weight onto the forward leg and then onto the rear leg.

Shift your weight completely, so that whichever leg you stand on supports you fully. Remember to let the foot of the leg that is not supporting you remain in partial contact with the floor for balance.

Be attentive to what you are doing as you shift your weight forward or backward. Are you comfortable throughout that movement? Could you stop and stand easily with your weight shifted one-quarter, one-half, or three-quarters of the way? Sense what happens in each foot as your weight rolls onto that foot or off of it. Can you move your head and eyes freely as you shift from one leg to the other?

Reverse your legs again. Continue to explore all that you do as you shift forward and backward. See if you can make that transition fluid and elegant. You might imagine that your pelvis is a pendulum, swinging through its arc and reversing smoothly.

4 Shift your weight onto your forward leg and stay there. See if you can stand securely with almost all of your weight on this forward leg. Remember to rest your hands on something to insure your balance. Be as comfortable as you can be while standing like this.

Now sense your rear leg and how that side is suspended from your pelvis. Can you sense the weight of that leg? If not, it means you are holding tighter than necessary either in that hip joint or in that side of your lower back.

Notice how the foot of your free leg touches the floor. Do you touch with your big toe mostly or with all the toes? Does your small toe touch the floor or is it in the air? What about the ball of your foot and the area at the base of your toes? How high is your heel lifted?

Gently move that free rear leg to alter the way your foot contacts the floor. As you have already discovered, your ability to move the free leg requires that you stand securely on the supporting leg. You might now find that gently moving the free rear leg helps you discover greater stability with the supporting leg.

5 Keep your weight on that same leg secure and steady. Remember to rest your hands on something for added balance.

Now simply swing your free rear foot forward to take a step. Touch that foot to the floor in front of you and leave that foot forward. But do so without shifting any weight onto it. Your weight stays on the same leg as in the previous movement.

Sense how this foot contacts the floor when it is in front. Do you touch the floor with your whole foot, with your heel only, or with your toes?

Some people touch the floor in front with only the toes, holding the heel in the air. That is especially common with women who often wear high heels or who studied ballet when they were young, but some men also touch the floor in front with the toes. Do that deliberately. Sense the effort required in the hip joint and the lower back on that side.

Continue to stand with all of your weight on the rear leg. Explore different ways of touching the floor with your forward foot. Touch the floor with your toes, your heel, more toward the inside of your foot or the outside of your foot.

As you explore touching the floor in different ways, see if you can eliminate any excess effort throughout that side. Sense the weight of your leg, your hip joint and pelvis, hanging downward. As always, breathe freely and be sure you do not fixate your head or eyes.

6   Continue to stand with all your weight on the same leg. Shift your free foot back again, to touch the floor behind you. Pause there for a moment to be sure you are standing securely and touching the floor easily.

Now swing that leg forward to touch the foot to the floor in front, easily. Then swing that leg backward again. And continue doing this. Let the leg that is swinging be completely free, pausing for a moment each time you touch with either the toes or the heel. Keep your weight securely on the other leg throughout the movement. See if you can eliminate any excess effort in either hip joint.

A moment ago, I suggested that you think of your pelvis as a pendulum, swinging smoothly to bring your weight over your forward foot or your rear foot. Now you can think of your leg as the pendulum, swinging forward and backward. The toe or heel can touch the floor for an instant at either end of the arc, then your leg smoothly swings again. Sense the weight of that pendulum as it swings.

Pause briefly.

7 Walk slowly. Sense any differences between the leg that has been supporting you and the leg that has been swinging forward and backward.

Can you detect any imbalance as you walk? Does one leg seem more secure, the other more mobile, from doing these movements on only one side?

Remember, learning occurs when we sense differences. Walk for a few moments and sense your legs and pelvis and everywhere. Compare your right leg and your left, and contrast how you are now with how you walk normally. If you like, walk in a small circle in each direction to see how you turn.

Walk and explore any differences in your legs for a few more moments. Be as aware of your supporting leg as you are of your stepping leg.

8 Again, stand where you can touch something for balance, with one leg in front of the other. Now stand with all your weight on the leg that had been swinging freely a moment ago. Be aware of how securely you stand on this leg.

With your weight on this leg, review steps 4, 5, and 6.

If you like, do this by imagining only. However, you will need to be especially attentive since walking is an extremely habitual act and the distinctions I am guiding you to make are relatively new to most people. An excellent way to learn is to imagine each movement as clearly as you can, then do it once or twice to compare how you move with what you imagined. This will help you to rediscover rapidly what you were learning while doing the movements on the opposite side.

9 Walk slowly again for a few moments. Sense how, during each step, you stand securely on one leg for an instant. At that moment, the opposite leg can be completely free, simply hanging

159

downward from your pelvis as it swings forward. Notice your feet as they contact the floor, how each foot rolls through that contact as your weight shifts. Be aware of your pelvis and how you move your pelvis steadily forward from one foot to the other.

Walk more slowly or a bit more quickly. Sense if your awareness changes as you alter the speed of your walking.

PART EIGHT *Lying on Your Back*

1 Lie on your back and rest for a moment. Begin to lengthen one side while you shorten your opposite side, as before.

Sense the movement all through your trunk, in your ribs all around, in your spine from your pelvis through to your neck. Again, notice how your ribs on one side squeeze together while on the opposite side they fan apart.

Pause.

2 Bend your legs and place your feet flat on the floor. Tilt your knees left and right.

Sense how tilting your knees rotates your pelvis and how that rotation is transmitted along your spine. What happens in your head? Do you turn in the direction toward which you are tilting your knees, in the opposite direction, or do you do something else? Just notice what happens spontaneously.

Continue to tilt your knees. Turn your head in the same direction, so that you are looking toward whichever side your knees are on. See if you can make this a simple, coordinated movement.

Pause.

Now tilt your knees left and right while intentionally turning your head in the opposite direction.

Continue to tilt your knees and roll your pelvis, and after every 2 or 3 movements reverse what you are doing with your head.

Compare these two variations. Sense what happens throughout your trunk, in your ribs on both sides and all around.

Rest for a moment. Extend your legs.

3 Simply turn your head left and right. The back of your head rolls on the floor and your chin moves toward one shoulder and then toward the other shoulder. As you roll your head, move your eyes and actively look left and right.

How far down your spine can you sense this movement? Are you aware of any movement between your shoulder blades, in your mid-back, your lower back, your pelvis?

Pause briefly.

4 Simultaneously turn your head left and right as you alternately lengthen one side and shorten the other. Do that a number of times.

Are you spontaneously coordinating these movements? If so, how? Are you turning your head toward the side that is becoming shorter or toward the side that is becoming longer?

Continue to turn your head as you lengthen and shorten your trunk. Sense how these movements connect or relate.

Pause.

5 Reverse the way you coordinate these movements. If you were looking toward the side that was becoming shorter, now look toward the side that is lengthening.

Is this easier, equivalent, or more difficult? Might there have been some reason you initially did it the other way? Do the movement this way a number of times.

6 Do 3 or 4 movements looking toward the side that shortens, then 3 or 4 movements looking toward the side that lengthens. Continue to change the pattern after every few movements.

Sense how you coordinate your head and pelvis. Your head, at one end of your spine, rolls and turns from side to side. At the opposite end of your spine, your pelvis tilts and slides on the floor. See if you can move your pelvis continuously, while reversing the direction of your head after every 3 or 4 movements.

Is one of these patterns easier or more fluid? Remember, what you do habitually will always seem easier at first. To sense accurately, you need to reduce any effort and become more aware.

This difference is rather subtle, yet one variation really is easier, due to reflexes that govern the muscle tone of head and neck movements. From my perspective, however, knowing the correct answer is not nearly as important as knowing how to seek your own answers. If I were to tell you which variation is easier, I would deprive you of the opportunity and motivation to inquire. In becoming more aware and learning for yourself, you gain self-reliance, self-esteem, and greater ability to learn in other situations.

If you continue to do these movements, gradually reducing any effort so that you can make more precise and subtle distinctions, you will discover which way is easier.

7 Rest. What are you aware of now? Notice how you contact the floor. Observe any images you have of yourself. Compare how you are now with how you were when you began this lesson.

Begin to roll slowly toward one side. Pause. And notice which side you were rolling toward. Did you choose this side only from habit, or was there some reason for the choice? As you roll toward one side and prepare to stand, notice whether you lengthen or shorten the side toward which you roll.

Roll toward one side and prepare to stand. Then roll toward the other side and prepare to stand. Do that rolling a few more times.

Sense how you roll your head and pelvis. Be aware of any lengthening or shortening on both sides.

Roll to either side and stand.

PART NINE *Walking, Swinging Your Arms, and Turning Your Head*

1 I encourage you to have fun with these final movements. Do them slowly or quickly, smoothly or awkwardly. Play.

Stand normally, with your legs parallel and at a comfortable distance from one another. Turn your head to look left and right. Let your arms hang or swing gently as you turn. Many times, turn left and right, moving freely everywhere.

What do you do as you turn your head? Can you sense any movement in your pelvis and hip joints? Do you shift your weight as you turn your head right and left?

2 Stand with one foot in front of the other, as it is when you have just taken a step. Shift your weight completely onto your rear leg, keeping your forward foot in contact with the floor for balance.

With all of your weight on your rear leg, turn your head from side to side. Let your arms swing left and right with your head. Make the movement smooth and fluid everywhere.

Sense the swinging in your head, shoulders, and arms as you look left and right. Notice how this involves your ribs, chest, and back, down to your pelvis and hip joints. See if you can balance securely on one leg, with your forward leg completely free.

If you feel unsteady and begin to lose your balance, turn your head and swing your arms more slowly, or make the movement smaller. Or just do it badly. If this seems awkward, consider how it was to be a young child first learning to stand and walk.

Pause for a moment.

3 Shift your weight onto your forward leg, leaving your rear foot in contact with the floor for balance.

Again, turn your head and swing your arms.

Remember, the more securely you stand on your forward leg, the more freely you can swing your arms and turn your head. Sense the range and quality of this movement.

Again, pause briefly.

4 Continue to stand with all of your weight on your forward leg.

Keep your face forward and begin to swing your arms again. You may want to look at whatever is in front of you, but be sure you do not stiffen your neck or fixate your head or eyes.

Notice how you swing your arms while facing forward. Do your arms seem to swing only from the shoulder joint, or can you sense some movement in your shoulder blades and collarbones?

*Part Nine
Step Four*

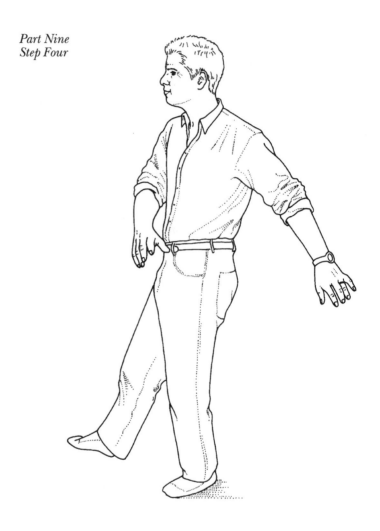

Swing your arms easily and see if you can move more freely everywhere.

5 As you continue to swing your arms, step forward with your rear leg but do not shift your weight onto it. Then move that leg back again.

Do that several times. While standing on one leg, continue to swing your arms as you bring the free leg forward and back. The foot of the free leg can touch the floor in front and behind, as you were doing a few moments ago, in Part Seven of this lesson.

6 The next time that foot is in front, shift your weight onto it. Continue to swing your arms while standing on this leg, with your head facing forward. Remember to keep your head and eyes free. And, as always, breathe easily.

Now swing the opposite foot forward and back, touching the floor with either the heel or the toes. Can you recall how your foot was swinging and touching the floor earlier, when you did that without swinging your arms?

A number of times, easily, swing your arms freely from side to side as you swing your leg forward and backward. Notice how you do this movement. Are you coordinating your leg and arms? How?

As your leg goes forward, do you move your arm on the same side forward, so that your leg and arm are moving in the same direction? Or do you move the opposite arm forward with your leg? Play with these two possibilities.

7 Shift your weight onto your opposite leg. Swing your arms again. At the same time, swing the leg that is now free to touch the floor in front and behind.

Again, coordinate your arms and leg. As your leg goes backward, do you swing the opposite arm backward? Or do you swing your arm and leg so that the arm on the side of the swinging leg moves in the same direction as the leg?

Do this movement a few times in each pattern. Remember to stand securely on the one leg and to keep your head free. Do what you can to eliminate excess effort everywhere.

Sense the difference between these two ways of swinging your arm and your leg. Does one pattern seem easier and more natural?

8 Stand for a moment with one leg in front of the other, as it would be if you had just taken a step, with your weight on the rear leg. Begin to swing your arms, moving your whole shoulder as you have been doing.

José was referred to me by an orthopedic surgeon following a back injury, his tenth in nearly 30 years of heavy construction work. After his previous injuries, José told me, physical therapy or chiropractic treatments had relieved his pain and enabled him to resume working. This time, however, he was still experiencing pain more than three months after the injury. Although he had returned to work, José was seeing his chiropractor at the end of each day and the chiropractor expected that regular treatments would be necessary for several more months. The orthopedic surgeon who made the referral and the insurance company that was paying the bill thought I might help José recover more quickly and completely.

From watching how José walked into my office, I could see distinct patterns of stiffening throughout his trunk. José learned quickly: After only a few sessions he reported that he was free from pain most of the time, although he still felt stiff and sore after prolonged sitting or heavy lifting.

In our seventh and eighth lessons, I helped José sense the movement of his pelvis while walking, using the same patterns as in this lesson. He immediately understood how he could use these movements to relieve tightness in his lower back. I suggested that he take a short walk and do that any time he sensed discomfort.

José turned, looked at me, and said, "You don't expect me to wiggle my butt in front of my work crew, do you?"

I looked him in the eyes and asked, "Would you rather wiggle your butt or be in pain?" Then I paused and observed him for a few moments. Before he said anything, I added, "Besides, you can do this movement so subtly that no one will notice. If you want to play with larger movements, you can simply walk out of their sight."

When I saw José a few days later he said that on the rare occasions when he still had any discomfort he just took a short walk. That was the tenth and last time I saw him. Just before leaving, he said that he felt better than he had in several decades. And, like many other people, José wanted to know why these lessons are not taught to everyone in schools.

After swinging your arms 2 or 3 times, shift your weight onto the forward leg. See if you can shift your weight without disrupting the movement in your arms.

Swing your arms 2 or 3 times, then step forward with your rear foot. See if you can step forward without disrupting the movement in your arms.

Continue to walk this way. The movement of your arms is continuous, and after every 2 or 3 movements of your arms, you either shift your weight forward or swing your rear foot forward.

Keep your head free, so that you can look around. Sense your balance on whichever is your supporting leg. See if you can eliminate any excess effort anywhere.

Pause and stand comfortably.

9 Now simply walk, slowly or more quickly, without thought or effort. Take large steps or small steps. Let your arms swing easily. Turn your head freely to look around.

Sense how you move your eyes and head, your arms and shoulders, your pelvis and hip joints, your legs and feet. Be as aware as you can be, while walking simply, easily.

Notice how you feel. Is this way of walking nice, pleasant, comfortable? How does this compare with your normal way of walking?

Learning and Life

Over 200 people gathered in Amherst, Massachusetts, in June 1980 for the beginning of a Feldenkrais Professional Training Program. Also present in the Hampshire College gymnasium were approximately 20 graduates of Moshe's San Francisco training, held 1975–1977, and six assistants who had studied with him in Tel Aviv since the 1960s. The Amherst course, the third and final training that Moshe personally taught, was scheduled to last four summers, nine weeks each session.

Moshe began that first day by saying, "I will learn more from this course than any of you." At the time he said that, Moshe was 76 and most of the students were in their twenties or thirties. Even so, I believe his expectation was sincere and, in the two summers before he became ill, fulfilled.

Moshe saw curiosity as a key to health, and he expressed his curiosity more freely than anyone I have ever known, other than a few young children whose parents wisely avoided inhibiting them. Yet he did not ask many questions. His curiosity about himself and everything around him was deeper than words, and he only asked questions when he sincerely needed to know something that he could not discover by observing and exploring on his own. In that way, he was like a healthy, preverbal child.

At the conclusion of the second summer in Amherst, Moshe asked me to join him in Washington, D.C., where he was to present a public workshop for 400 people. We stayed with Allison Rapp and Roger Miller, graduates of the San Francisco course, who lived in the northwest part of the city. The day before the workshop, Moshe wanted to rest at the house alone, so I accompanied Allison on a series of errands while Roger went to set up the sound system in the ballroom at the Hilton, where the three-day workshop was to be held. After dinner that evening, Moshe began to describe the things he had discovered while looking through cabinets and drawers all over the house. Allison leaned over to me and whispered, "I hope he didn't go through my old checkbooks."

After childhood, most learning involves discovering new ways to do something you already know how to do. If you know only one way to do something, you have no real choice regarding the action. Either you do it, or not. Learning a second way of doing something frees you from this compulsive all-or-nothing pattern. To have only two options is still a rather limited way of functioning, however. Once acquired, a third option is truly liberating, since it generally enables you to begin to discover new alternatives spontaneously. That, according to Moshe, is the sign of fully human activity. In Lesson Six, *Elegant Walking*, you learned three ways to move your pelvis with each step, and if you review that lesson you may devise numerous variations.

As an example from my own experience, I like to cite the way I cross my legs while sitting. When I began with the Feldenkrais Method, I noticed that I habitually crossed my left leg over the right so that the left ankle was on the right thigh. I occasionally crossed my right leg over the left, yet I typically did so with the thighs close together. Curious about that pattern, I began to play with it. Each time I noticed that I was in the habitual position I would change to the symmetrical variation. Now I can cross either leg tightly or more openly, or I can sit with both feet on the floor, all with comparable ease and freedom.

Of the thousands of movements that anyone is capable of making, each of us adopts a relatively small repertoire. With greater awareness and curiosity about yourself, you can discover new possibilities for everything you do. If your current way of doing something is ineffective, especially if it involves pain, you will then be able to find more satisfying alternatives.

169

A particularly good time to review these lessons, in whole or part, is just before some familiar exercise or activity. If you bring an attitude of awareness and comfort with you onto the golf course or tennis court, you will certainly enhance your enjoyment of the game. My students often report that their skill and scores also improve, sometimes dramatically. You might devise ways to integrate these lessons into aerobics classes, using exercise equipment, or other fitness activities. If your instructors want to know why you sometimes disobey exhortations to increase your speed or effort, blame me and tell them about the Feldenkrais Method.

Applying the lessons in these ways will help you avoid the tendency to compartmentalize, which is a major obstacle to learning. I have seen people show real grace and skill on the tennis court or dance floor yet move clumsily and ineffectively everywhere else. Many students of yoga, T'ai Chi, or other disciplines move beautifully during their practice, but forget everything when they return to the street. Conversely, compartmentalizing our ways of acting can be healthy and appropriate: Some young girls who take ballet classes continue to walk with their hip joints turned out, and I have seen many adult women with hip, knee, or lower back problems who describe having done that as young ballerinas.

I often advise my students to make simple movements, such as the ones in these lessons, while engaging in other activities—and a few people actually listen and follow that suggestion. One who did was Linda, an artist and massage therapist who used to come to me for both classes and individual lessons. When waiting for an appointment one day, she was sitting on the floor of my office reading while moving. Furthermore, instead of doing only small movements, she was tilting her legs and rolling freely from side to side. Linda was moving so beautifully that for several minutes I watched from the doorway, delighted, to verify that she was turning the pages at regular intervals and actually reading. I was especially impressed because she was not reading a magazine or romance novel but something rather demanding—Moshe's book, *The Elusive Obvious*.

The most exciting aspect of the Feldenkrais Method for me is its promise of continued learning throughout life. I have done some of these lessons dozens, even hundreds, of times. Provided that I am really doing the lesson, not mindlessly repeating the movements, I learn and improve each time. That attitude seems to extend more and more to almost everything I do, and each year I feel younger and more alive.

A few years ago, I was on the faculty of a Feldenkrais Professional Training segment in Brisbane, Australia. The senior trainer for the segment, Mark Reese, asked me to teach a series of Awareness Through Movement lessons in the sitting position, several of which are variations of the lessons in this book. I taught one of these lessons every few days. On some of the days when I was not teaching, Mark presented a series of rather challenging lessons that involved reorganizing the legs and hip joints to squat on the heels in different ways. Toward the end of the month-long training, I sat on a wooden stool one day to think about the next lesson I was going to teach. When I began subtly to tilt my pelvis, I sensed an extraordinary freedom and elasticity in my hip joints, deep in my pelvis. The experience was so different from anything I had known previously that I jumped up to see if the stool was rocking on an uneven place in the floor. It was not the stool. With my new awareness of my hip joints, I began to discover not only greater freedom when sitting, but also increased skill and enjoyment in walking, dancing, and other activities.

Life does not always afford the opportunity for active learning, however. Sacrifice and struggle may be unavoidable at times. Opportunities to truly value comfort may be rare and easily overlooked. We all know how to lose ourselves amidst our continual everyday distractions.

You can prepare for trying or difficult times by taking the opportunity to learn now. Even more importantly, you can cultivate the attitude of continuing to learn. Any time you experience stress, injury, or illness, this attitude and enhanced awareness will help you recover more quickly and completely.

The major obstacles to this organic way of learning fall into two categories: habit and social pressures. Habits are essential to life. The simplest acts would take impossibly long without the streamlining effect of habit. Most people believe that habits exert some magical force that makes change very difficult, but the Feldenkrais Method proves otherwise. It is only when we try to change habits through force of will alone that we struggle and usually fail. When you clearly experience increasing skill and comfort with a different way of acting, even the most deeply rooted habit can be replaced instantaneously. Habits are only dysfunctional when they involve some discomfort or pain, but any pain can serve to remind and motivate you to learn a more effective alternative. In fact, most of us already know alternatives, and with awareness these can be readily accessed and integrated.

Social pressures may involve an actual expression of disapproval by someone, or may be only your internalized concern or anxiety. A number of people have said to me: "I can't move like that during a meeting"; "My wife complains if I'm doing these movements in nice restaurants"; or, "If people see me tilting my pelvis, they'll think I'm out looking for sex."

For years I have responded to these comments by emphasizing that these movements really are most effective when done with the least effort, minimally. The benefits come from your awareness, not from stretching or exercising muscles. You can make these movements so small and subtle that they are completely invisible to anyone around you, even to your spouse at your side or your friends around the room. In doing that, you will often benefit more than from moving more actively or forcefully.

I encourage you, however, to sometimes play with larger movements and different possibilities, even if other people notice. In addition to the benefits of moving, this will help you overcome excessive or unreasonable inhibitions. Most of us are oversocialized, and we suffer in various ways from placing other people's opinions above our own comfort. If someone does comment or criticize, you can describe what you are doing and help the person learn to be more aware and move more comfortably. He or she will probably be extremely grateful.

Now, so you will be fully human, I offer a third alternative. If you are bending, twisting, leaning, circling your pelvis, or doing anything for your own benefit or enjoyment, and you notice someone staring, you can do what Moshe sometimes did: turn toward the person and stick out your tongue.

Toward a Science of Health

The Feldenkrais Method is, in Moshe's words, "somewhere between intuition and future scientific gospel."

As a scientist, Moshe was an empiricist who valued observation and experimentation while challenging theories and abstractions. He was also a generalist, proud to have earned a Doctorate of Science, D.Sc., rather than a Ph.D. in any specialized field. With Frédéric Joliot-Curie at the Sorbonne, Moshe helped design and build several Van de Graaff generators and equipment for research into radioactivity, employing his training in mechanical and electrical engineering, physics, and mathematics. While working for the British Admiralty during World War II, he helped develop sonar and underwater detection devices. Moshe also studied neurophysiology, ethology, cybernetics, and other disciplines, and was extremely interested in spiritual and psychological practices, both Western and Eastern.

Over several decades of studying and teaching judo, Moshe applied his scientific training and observational abilities to analyzing the mechanics that make various judo moves effective. Through doing this, he developed ways to understand healthy, efficient movement generally, for any person or activity. Moshe was also inspired and influenced by observing babies, and he recognized that babies spontaneously move in ideal ways. As I discussed in the first chapter, Moshe had severely injured his left knee as a young man and he reinjured that knee while in England in the 1940s. After being told he needed surgery and might never walk normally, he applied his scientific training, judo experience, and insights into how babies learn to crawl and walk—and he learned to walk so skillfully that he never had surgery and was able to resume his judo.

I often heard people ask Moshe to compare his methods with physical therapy or chiropractic treatments, or with alternatives such as yoga, acupressure, Rolfing, or the Alexander Technique. Other people wanted his opinion of different spiritual practices or systems of psychotherapy. To questions of this kind, Moshe usually responded, "My work is more fundamental."

Advocates of particular approaches often resented Moshe's statement, dismissing it, and him, as arrogant and egotistical. Those who continued to listen, however, sometimes understood that he was referring to his quest for fundamental insights into health and human behavior. As a scientist, Moshe was not content with being able to help people; he wanted to understand how people heal and learn with any approach or treatment, or spontaneously.

When asked about his work and way of thinking, Moshe liked to say that his genius was an ability to "make the abstract concrete." The Feldenkrais Method demonstrates this by integrating many disciplines and all aspects of life.

Physical Experience

As "human" beings, we are animals and physical beings also, and laws of motion and mechanics apply universally. In humans and machines, inefficient movements involve friction, produce heat, and eventually lead to problems. When learning to move as babies, each of us moved efficiently—we lacked the strength to do otherwise. As we grew and gained strength, however, we lost that natural awareness and skill, at least partially.

Rosa had injured her shoulders and upper back while working as a supervisor at a produce canning factory. She had undergone chiropractic treatment for several months after her injury, followed by a few months of physical therapy, before an orthopedic surgeon sent her to me. As we talked at the start of her first lesson, I sat next to Rosa, gently lifted her right arm to shoulder height, and then released it—and the arm remained in the air. I asked, "Rosa, do you sense your arm?" She did not, and was surprised when I asked her to turn and look. The muscles in Rosa's shoulder were so tight that, whether her arm was lifted or hanging freely at her side, she could not sense anything other than her pain.

I worked with Rosa lying in different positions, sitting, standing, walking, with her eyes open and looking at her arms, and with her eyes closed. In each lesson, we explored additional ways for her to be more aware of gravity, how she responded or resisted, and the effort involved. After only six lessons, the insurance administrator sent Rosa back to the orthopedic surgeon for a final medical evaluation. When she saw the doctor, Rosa declared that the six lessons with me had helped more than all previous treatments combined.

If someone is completely relaxed and you lift and then release one hand, the hand will fall just like the apple that inspired Isaac Newton. If the hand stays in the air, even for a moment, it indicates that muscles are working. While Rosa's condition was more extreme than most, each of us tenses and resists gravity in various ways, all of them futile. Inefficient movements and disturbed biomechanics are present in every case of back pain, arthritis, or other musculoskeletal problems.

Relative to gravity and other forces, structural support for any movement comes from the skeleton. While we all have seen models or pictures of the skeleton, we sense our own skeletal structures only incompletely. Awareness of the skeleton must come from experience, not from studying anatomy books: I have worked with doctors and physical therapists who know theoretical anatomy much more thoroughly than I, but who have never clearly sensed their own hip joints or clavicles. Evoking a more complete and accurate sense of one's skeleton is an important theme in most Awareness Through Movement lessons. You may want to review the six lessons in this book while being especially attentive to your skeleton and gravity, and you will experience significant benefits if you do.

Our upright human stance raises our center of gravity higher than in other animals, and people sometimes believe that back pain is the unavoidable result. That notion, from a functional perspective, is silly. When one sits or stands efficiently, the head and shoulders are over the center of gravity in the pelvis and the base of support at the feet. Gravity and other forces are transmitted directly through the bones, leaving muscles free and loose and able to move in any direction. Engineers describe this high center of gravity as a dynamic, unstable equilibrium. As Moshe understood, we evolved for and through movement.

Physiological Matters

Muscles can contract, or they can stop contracting, which allows them to lengthen, and every joint in the skeleton has muscles arranged in pairs or groups so that as one contracts its opposite lengthens. These opposite muscles are labeled antagonists, which suggests internal resistance. When one moves efficiently, however, as each muscle contracts its opposite lengthens simultaneously and both muscles have relatively equal tone. Any sense of resistance or internal opposition indicates some disturbance from this ideal. If you are fighting against yourself, you lose.

Yet most systems of exercise focus on specific muscles or muscle groups while ignoring their opposites. Of the thousands of people I have worked with, not one of those who did sit-ups—like Sylvia, whose story I told at the introduction to Lesson One—was aware of the back muscles lengthening as the abdominal muscles contract. Furthermore, many people do sit-ups while straining and holding their breath, which restricts movement in both the back and abdomen. In Lesson One, *Bending and Breathing,* you learned to breathe and sense the movement all around, and this awareness makes sit-ups or any other exercise more enjoyable and beneficial.

Commonly, people are taught to stretch after exercise, yet stretching without awareness can also be counterproductive. When stretched with excess force, muscles respond by contracting, and every muscle fiber contains a stretch-reflex nerve receptor that regulates this. The stretch-reflex is why people repeat the same stretches regularly yet rarely realize any lasting improvement. As you learn to be more aware and move more skillfully, you quiet and reset the stretch receptors and allow permanent lengthening. I hope you discovered this with the six lessons. You can verify this fact and enhance these benefits by reviewing the lessons more slowly and comfortably.

A muscle is strongest when it can fully contract from its greatest resting length in the least time, and this can only occur when the opposite muscle harmoniously lengthens from complete contraction. Muscles are simultaneously stronger and more relaxed when one is aware and moving efficiently; you may have noticed this after the lessons as a sense of being taller or lighter. For their size, children are much stronger than adults, and their strength comes from moving efficiently as they play spontaneously, not from doing structured, repetitive exercises.

Awareness and efficient movement facilitate recovery from any injury, illness, disease, or difficulty, while stiffness or immobility exacerbates most problems. All physiological matters involve movement: circulation requires not only the heart muscle, but movement everywhere; in fact, some textbooks refer to the leg muscles as an "auxiliary heart," and anyone with swelling of the feet or ankles, or edema, can benefit from moving those areas more freely. Respiration can involve moving all the muscles of the trunk, as you experienced in Lesson Four, *Uninhibited Breathing*. To breathe with the chest or diaphragm only is actually more difficult, but habitual for many people. Digestion uses muscles that line the stomach and intestines, and this action is affected by the muscles around the trunk. The immune, nervous, and endocrine systems depend upon movement and muscular action for the flow of lymph, cerebrospinal fluid, and other materials.

Research is beginning to verify the importance of aware, efficient movement for all healing.

Neurological Organization

Moshe insisted that any attempt to understand or influence human behavior must respect the overall functioning of the brain. Language, culture, consciousness, and all that we think of as uniquely human evolved rather recently, and these capacities represent a relatively small fraction of neurological activity. The primary functions of the brain involve more basic biological processes that maintain life and insure survival.

Fundamental to all neurological behaviors is creating invariance, constructing a stable representation from the chaos of complex and continually changing sensory inputs. While some people describe the newborn infant's brain as a "tabula rasa," a blank slate upon which the world writes, this can be true only with respect to content. The process of constructing invariance and making sense of the world requires sophisticated innate neurological capacities, such as Noam Chomsky postulated for grammar. Gerald Edelman, who received the 1972 Nobel Prize in Physiology or Medicine, presents a model for this in his books *Neural Darwinism* (Basic Books, 1987) and *Bright Air, Brilliant Fire* (Basic Books, 1992).

We commonly speak and think about having five senses, yet the inputs to the central nervous system overwhelmingly involve the experience of the body in space and in action. This means that the proprioceptive and kinesthetic sense, sometimes called the sixth sense, is first in many ways: your ability to see, hear, touch, taste, and smell depends on how you move. Where movement is limited or disturbed, sensation is distorted or disappears altogether. As each of us knows, when we touch or are being touched, sensation fades while we are motionless and increases with changing contact. Scientists have confirmed this in the laboratory in many ways, for every sense. For example, when researchers use curare to paralyze the muscles that move the eyes, vision ceases within a few moments unless objects within the field of vision move or the research subject moves his or her whole head.

The early hours, days, months, even years, of a child's life are mostly dedicated to this process of creating invariance. This process continues throughout one's life, yet it is so thorough and fundamental that we only recognize it under extreme circumstances, as when sight is gained by someone who was blind from birth. In each case where this has been documented, learning to see was a slow, tedious process that continued to be unreliable for many years. The brain, having organized independent of visual information, was only able to make sense of patterns of light after repeated experiences of correlating what was seen with touch, taste, smell, sound, and, especially, movement. Oliver Sacks and other scientists have written about the physical, perceptual, and psychological struggles these individuals experience.

Anatomy and physiology textbooks typically contain a diagram of a homunculus, or "little man," the body as represented on the sensory cortex of the brain. This homunculus is significantly different from the body seen objectively, with such deviations as lips and thumbs larger than the trunk. These representations are unique to each individual and change with experience. For example, there will be more detail for the fourth finger of anyone who plays a musical instrument than for someone who never develops comparable dexterity. To test this hypothesis, Eric Kandel and scientists at Columbia University mapped the electrical activity for areas of the cortex representing the fingers in adult monkeys. They then trained the monkeys to do specific movements that involved only a few fingers. After three months, the areas that represented the active fingers were substantially larger than before the experiment, while the cortex area for the other fingers was relatively smaller. This evidence that we act in accordance with unique, learned, changing cortical maps illustrates the fundamental importance of the theoretical insights Moshe recognized and applied—insights that are generally ignored.

Another example is the Weber-Fechner Law, first described in the 1860s. The Weber-Fechner law says that the ability to detect any change in a stimulus varies in direct proportion to the intensity of the stimulus. This is considered a law, not merely a hypothesis or theory, since it has been proved true for all perceptual activity, with no exceptions. This means that someone carrying a heavy weight—Moshe would use the exaggerated example of a piano—will not detect any change if a fly lands on it or takes off again, while someone holding only a feather can sense the weight of the fly. When standing outside on a sunny day, you cannot notice any increased light from a candle behind you, but in a dark room you could read after lighting that same candle.

The Weber-Fechner law is the reason I advised you repeatedly to use minimal effort while doing the lessons: By reducing your effort, you simultaneously learn to sense more accurately and to move more skillfully. If you want to detect whether a fly lands or takes off from a feather you are holding, you will do better if you are aware and holding the feather lightly, since excess effort in your fingers, hand, arm, or anywhere will interfere with your ability to sense. As this shows, moving and sensing are inseparable neurologically and therefore in every act—but not, unfortunately, in the way we commonly think and speak.

Moshe described one way he tested this for himself: While resting his forearm on a table he took hold of a hammer by the end of the handle. With the hammer on the table at a 90-degree angle to his arm, he began to turn his hand over and back, so that the heavy end of the hammer made an arc over his hand. He did that each day for some minutes. Every few days Moshe added a bit of lead to the head of the hammer, with each addition calculated to be small enough that he would not detect any difference in the weight being lifted. After six months the hammer weighed over six kilograms, and was so heavy that most people could not even lift it in that position. Yet Moshe twiddled it easily from side to side, and he achieved that without ever feeling that he was doing hard work or exercising.

From a functional perspective, every act involves moving, sensing, feeling, and thinking, all highly organized and integrated. While the brain is often described in terms of specific parts, layers, hemispheres, or control centers, any excitation or specialization occurs within the context of whole brain activity. Recent research, especially that using positron-emission tomography, PET scans, supports the functional, holistic neurological insights Moshe insisted upon over 50 years ago.

Emotional/Psychological Concerns

While living in England during World War II, Moshe spent time at the Institute for Visiting Scholars along with other European scientists who had fled the Nazis. In the evenings, residents of the Institute would share their ideas with one another. Whenever the subject was psychology, Moshe would sit quietly in the back of the room until he could no longer contain his frustration: "You keep talking about the inferiority complex, but you never describe the person who feels inferior. Was he short, ugly, stupid? Did he have a small penis? Maybe he had good reason to feel inferior. How can you go on talking as if this inferiority complex is some kind of thing apart from a real, unique person?"

Psychotherapeutic approaches commonly focus on content and interpretation, while the Feldenkrais Method views psychological concerns in terms of concrete processes and behaviors. Without any psychological probing, my students often gain insight into their emotional experiences, frequently at the moment of discovering that some problem or limitation has disappeared, as if spontaneously. People sometimes laugh, cry, or express other emotions during a Feldenkrais lesson, and those feelings can be integrated into the learning experience.

All emotions—joy or love as much as rage or fear—always involve changes in breathing and muscular activity in the chest, neck, and elsewhere. Moshe particularly objected to the idea that emotions are somehow stored, repressed, or pent-up in the body. Emotional outbursts of the kind that are often described as pent-up can be better understood as indicating ways in which the person does not know how to act more skillfully. Someone who has never learned to modulate the expression of anger may explode with inappropriate rage, but that does not mean the anger was trapped like water behind a dam. Whatever one has learned or not learned, behavior occurs in the present.

You can test this quite simply: Recall the movements you learned in Lesson One, *Bending and Breathing*, and begin to do them, minimally. Breathe out and gently bend, then straighten as you breathe in. You might also recall Lesson Four, *Uninhibited Breathing*, and think about how your trunk is like a balloon, taking shape as you fill with air, then flexing or folding as you release the air. Sense the movement in your pelvis and upper chest as you continue to breathe easily and make some minimal movement. Now recall some emotionally intense moment, vividly, and reconstruct that experience for a few moments. Notice if doing this disrupts the way you are breathing and moving.

As you learn to breathe and act more effectively, you can express and resolve emotional concerns in ways that increasingly serve to realize your intentions. That learning can occur through behavioral approaches, with the verbal methods of conventional psychotherapies, or along with other experiences. When you learn to move more skillfully in the controlled, comfortable conditions of a Feldenkrais lesson, you can then generalize your experience to other situations. You can learn to breathe easily and feel good even while talking about or to your boss or mother.

As babies, each of us knew the experience of being omnipotent, the absolute center of the universe around whom all revolves. As we grew and became increasingly conditioned by society, however, most of us learned to feel relatively insignificant. We are psychologically most healthy when we can simultaneously acknowledge our omnipotence and our insignificance. Then we have the greatest freedom to act voluntarily, without any compulsiveness. For Moshe, this defined mature behavior.

Mental Understandings

Moshe hated to have his work viewed just in terms of the body, and he berated people who said that the goal of the Feldenkrais Method was only to relieve pain or improve movement. In response to a question about the value of becoming more flexible, he once said, "Was Einstein flexible? Was Newton flexible? We're interested in flexible minds, not just flexible bodies."

For Moshe, "Real thinking leads to new ways of acting." Functional thinking does not occur in words, generally, and we restrict our freedom and creativity when we confuse thinking and talking. We need to talk, socially and to ourselves, to express our ideas and construct our models of the world, but we also need to be able to stop the internal dialogue, which Moshe sometimes derided as "cerebration with words" or "mental masturbation." Words can be terribly inadequate for communication, although for most purposes they are the best we can do.

Like healthy movement of any kind, skillful thinking can reverse direction free of any constraints or compulsiveness. Moshe insisted that intellectual mastery of any subject involves the ability to present all points of view so authoritatively that the most ardent proponents agree that their cause has been furthered. He demonstrated this in the Amherst training, mentioned at the start of the preceding chapter, with a detailed talk about how Andrew Carnegie had been a great benefactor of humanity. Carnegie funded libraries and educational institutions around the world, and Moshe received two Carnegie scholarships during his years of study in Paris. Even as several students with strong leftist political views became quite enraged, Moshe continued to praise Carnegie's contributions. The following day Moshe spent almost as much time arguing that Carnegie had been a menace to humanity, a true robber baron who abused his workers, despoiled the environment, and produced tremendous suffering along with his steel.

Another way that Moshe challenged his students to really learn was by refusing to allow us to take notes during the Amherst training. He encouraged us to write during the breaks and in the evenings, to form study groups and share our insights, but he insisted that most note-taking reinforces mental laziness and insecurity. At one point, when a group of students persisted in taking notes, Moshe walked out of the room, announcing that he would not continue the program if the students refused to trust him. He was much more interested in teaching us to think than in simply training a new generation of Feldenkrais practitioners.

Real thinking—functional, appropriate, integrating all aspects of experience—is one of the greatest expressions of a creative life.

Spiritual Orientation

When he visited New York City, Moshe often stayed at Jane Parsons's apartment on Central Park West. I was there with him one evening when he began to read a popular book on spiritual development that had been prominently placed next to the kitchen table. Like many similar books, this one talked about love, forgiveness, compassion, the soul, and God, with a number of affirmations and exercises for readers to practice. After reading for a while, Moshe put the book down, shook his head slowly from side to side, and muttered, "Poverty of spirit."

We are impoverished when any aspect of experience is neglected. Books on spirituality and psychological growth present myths, symbols, and metaphors, many wonderful images, while generally ignoring or denying sensory-motor experience. Even when talking about or advocating awareness, which such approaches often do, most remain abstract. While a number of religious traditions, ancient and modern, use walking as a meditative practice, they typically do so in formal, ritualized ways.

Whatever one believes or practices, we are bodily, physical beings. The path to the infinite and eternal begins here and now, in the way we breathe, sit, walk, and function at every moment. The same word, *grace*, describes both spiritual attainment and aesthetically satisfying movement, and I find this significant and appropriate. Awareness heals and reawakens one's sense of wholeness, of being fully alive, which is the essence of spiritual experience.

Aware moving can evoke deeply meditative experiences, as you may discover if you review the lessons in this book with sufficient care and delicacy. If you learn to do Lesson Six, *Elegant Walking*, as slowly as you can, balancing securely on each leg, shifting your weight effortlessly, swinging your arms harmoniously, all without disturbing your breathing, you may experience greater stillness and inner peace than through any motionless meditation. I encourage you to explore that.

Social Variables

To a much greater extent than we commonly realize, sex, class, race, and ethnicity influence the way we sit and walk, how we gesture, our muscle tone and behavior. Careful observers can often use these clues to identify specific aspects of a person's background and life experience. Skillful actors both understand these factors and know how to re-create them. As you become more aware, you can learn to move and express yourself with much greater range and freedom than you currently know.

Among the questions Moshe asked people who came to him for lessons, often before inquiring about their difficulty, were what job the person held and what he or she did for recreation. We adapt our movement patterns and physical structures to the activities we commonly perform. A construction worker or professional athlete needs to learn ways of moving that would be inappropriate for someone who sits at a computer all day, and vice versa.

In large workshops, Moshe delighted in using Awareness Through Movement to demonstrate our natural sociability. He developed a number of lessons that conclude with people rolling freely from side to side. To prevent collisions, individuals who are close together need to coordinate their rolling. With sufficient awareness and time, people spontaneously discover a shared rhythm, and whole rows begin to roll harmoniously without any drumming, spoken direction, or other external regulation.

All social behavior depends on awareness, or suffers for its absence. We stop at red lights only when we see them, we help our neighbors only when we acknowledge their needs. With reduced awareness, we become increasingly selfish and life is much less pleasant for everyone. In learning to be more aware, through the six lessons in this book and in any other way, you benefit yourself, everyone with whom you interact, and society as a whole.

Love is impossible without respect. When unaware, however, we cannot respect others, or even ourselves. Through enhancing awareness we gain greater capacity to love.

Environmental Considerations

Our physical structures are intimately attuned to our environment, having evolved through millions of years with gravity, the ground beneath us, and the air around us. Humans raised in space or on another planet would be taller, shorter, or rounder, according to conditions there, as demonstrated by the rapid loss of bone and muscle mass in orbiting astronauts. Our eyes and ears evolved to perceive light and sound vibrations of the particular frequencies transmitted through the air on our planet Earth. If there were no light, we would not have eyes.

To survive, we need to accurately perceive our environment, and our physical structure reflects this. We evolved with eyes, ears, and nostrils in the head, at the top of the body, these paired organs parallel to the horizon to allow us to perceive distant stimuli and to orient appropriately. Mobility of the eyes and head can be essential for survival, and when we move efficiently, with the large muscles in the pelvis supplying the power and the skeleton supporting the weight, the head is always free to scan the environment and initiate action.

How one relates to the environment is an important indicator of health. When healthy, we are naturally curious, as children demonstrate, and we continually observe the world around us, although we may not be aware of doing so. Someone in pain is much less attentive and often immobilizes the head and eyes, at times reaching out to touch a wall, chair, street sign, or other object for the contact and orientation that is otherwise lacking.

As individuals and collectively, we can learn to value our contact with the environment as a fundamental aspect of our human nature. Thus, learning to be more aware as we breathe, sit, and walk may help us gain the wisdom to save our planet from further degradation.

Developmental Perspectives

Awareness of how people grow and change throughout their lives is fundamental to the Feldenkrais Method. Moshe was extremely critical of static notions in any form or context.

From birth to death, one changes continuously, and many problems result from trying to ignore or deny change. Every cell in the body dies and is replaced over a period of hours, days, or weeks. While conventional concerns focus primarily on undesired changes, most biological processes are reversible under the right conditions. Even the shape of the bones changes as calcium is deposited and taken up again, which is how exercise can prevent or reverse osteoporosis. As long as one is alive, one can learn and heal every day—physically, neurologically, psychologically, mentally, and spiritually.

In January 1981, *Smithsonian* magazine published an article which described how Moshe was able to help children who had cerebral palsy. The story, by esteemed science writer Albert Rosenfeld, and the prestige of *Smithsonian* attracted considerable attention. I was working as Moshe's appointment secretary the following summer and was contacted by parents and grandparents from around the country who wanted to bring children to Moshe in Amherst. My job, I soon discovered, was to say no to most of these requests, as politely and helpfully as possible. I sometimes described myself as a "disappointment secretary."

A number of adults, some quite elderly, also wanted lessons with Moshe. At first I thought to favor the children who had their whole lives in front of them. When I asked Moshe about that, however, he told me I was wrong to make any assumptions based on age: "An older person may be able to use the wisdom of experience to learn much more quickly than even a child. And with that life experience, the older person may then take what has been learned and do something that will enrich all humanity. You can never know. Some people are senile at twenty." Desire to learn was Moshe's main concern, and can be independent of age.

In a world of constant change, Moshe insisted that "There is nothing permanent about our behavior unless our beliefs make it so."

The Feldenkrais Method

Common concepts and conventional treatments focus on specifics, as if people can be divided into parts or levels: physical, neurological, psychological, mental, social, spiritual. These divisions are abstract and artificial, however, occurring in words only. The world and our experience are complex, continuous, simultaneous, multidimensional.

Moshe called his work Functional Integration to acknowledge the pattern that connects all aspects of life. He chose the name Awareness Through Movement for his group lessons to emphasize the fact that healing and rediscovering wholeness require awareness. Life is a process, and Moshe recognized that every aspect of that process involves movement. By improving the quality of movement, the Feldenkrais Method enhances all aspects of life.

Awareness Heals

The Feldenkrais Method incorporates a way of thinking that is, in the opinion of many, simultaneously new and intuitively true. Instead of viewing people objectively, from the outside, Moshe discovered a rigorously functional perspective which recognizes how each individual uniquely experiences and makes sense of the world. Philosophers have discussed similar concepts in various ways, as phenomenology, existentialism, experientialism, or constructivism, and the Feldenkrais Method makes these abstract ideas concrete and useful.

Organic Learning

Lift one hand, hold it so you can look into your palm, and begin to move your fingers, gently. Observe what happens in your fingers, hand, arm, shoulder, and everywhere. Sense the ease and range of movement, the weight of your fingers and changing pull of gravity as you move. Now, slowly, bring your hand to your face to touch your lips, nose, chin, and cheeks. Notice the contact, both in your fingers and in your face. Continue exploring in this way for a few moments, perhaps closing your eyes and reflecting on the complexity of this simple, everyday act.

As a baby, you devoted countless hours and days to exploring in these ways. Before learning to walk or talk, each of us had to learn to move and sense our hands, mouths, and feet—and this is how. Moshe called this "organic learning," to differentiate it from academic learning, social learning, or related activities of older children and adults.

To appreciate organic learning more fully, recall some time or situation in which you observed a baby, perhaps your child or grandchild. Babies learn by playfully exploring and imitating, motivated mostly by innate curiosity and guided always by exquisite awareness of comfort. While a newborn baby cannot walk into a restaurant and order breakfast, we can view turning to the nipple and taking it in the mouth, the reflexive acts of rooting and sucking, as first approximations of those adult abilities. After two to four months, each baby begins to put fingers, toes, and anything within reach, including food, into the mouth. In doing this, the baby learns simultaneously to sense and coordinate muscles, orient hand and mouth in space, identify and manipulate objects, form and realize intentions. Random or reflexive movements, repeated sufficiently, are distinguished and refined into voluntary acts. This spontaneous, self-organizing process is so elegant and reliable that 99.99 percent of babies succeed in learning to walk and talk, the most profound and powerful learning of our lives.

Through experience and organic learning, each of us actively makes sense of the world, integrating genetic factors with environmental influences. Most people, including scientists, presume some genetic cause whenever children and parents or siblings develop similar diseases or difficulties. As we have all observed, however, as children grow they imitate their parents' postures, gestures, attitudes, and dietary preferences, usually without knowing they are doing so. Asthma, arthritis, and other conditions may involve genetic predispositions, yet organic learning affects how, when, or if problems develop. In acknowledging the fundamental fact and importance of organic learning, we may be able to resolve the debate about nature versus nurture.

If you set aside conditioned or preconceived notions, you will begin to see organic learning everywhere, in yourself and everyone else. Moshe found, and I agree, that one of the best ways to understand this process is to observe children respectfully, to

189

respond and interact without teaching or treating or otherwise interfering. For many adults, simply being present and aware is uncomfortable, however, especially when a child seems to be experiencing some difficulty.

Heather was six years old when her mother, Sandra, first brought her to me. At the age of three months, Heather had been diagnosed as profoundly retarded with hypotonic cerebral palsy. In periodic evaluations over the years, doctors had said there were few prospects for any progress. The first time I saw Heather, she could not crawl or independently roll, she communicated only minimally, and she expressed little curiosity about the world.

When we began, Heather, like many children labeled autistic or profoundly retarded, would sometimes press her fingers forcefully into her eyes or bite her fingers so hard she left deep teeth marks. Doctors and therapists had labeled these behaviors "self-stimulating" and instructed Sandra to stop Heather from doing them. Sandra had tried, but telling Heather, "No! Stop biting," or attempting to pull the fingers out of her mouth or eyes was futile and counterproductive: Heather bit harder, Sandra felt frustrated and inadequate, and their communication was completely disrupted.

Sandra was disturbed by the doctor's advice and wanted to know what I thought was best for Heather. I helped Sandra observe more insightfully to consider what Heather might be experiencing, how she acquired those behaviors, and why they persisted. For Heather, it seemed to me, biting her fingers was simple and familiar, a reliable way to recover a feeling of order and security that must have provided a needed contrast to the confusion and frustration she often felt. Before biting her fingers, Heather would stiffen and hold her breath, and whenever I saw her do that I gently helped mobilize her neck and chest so that she could breathe more easily and move more comfortably. Heather began to improve from our first lesson. With my guidance, Sandra soon learned to identify these behaviors and help Heather in these ways. In just a few months, Heather stopped biting her fingers or pressing her eyes, easily outgrowing her long-standing habit.

Much of what I do with Heather or other children looks like play, and she often laughs or otherwise indicates how much she enjoys the learning we do together. For me, however, each lesson presents the continual challenge to be aware of what she is experiencing so that I can assist her in realizing her intentions. Heather and I have been learning together for six years, once or twice each week at times, but often skipping several weeks or months. Today Heather is alert and active, plays with dolls and toys, rolls and pulls herself along the floor, and communicates her needs through specific signs and sounds. She especially enjoys horseback riding. Family members or friends who knew her from before sometimes refer to her as "the new Heather."

Like all healthy children, Heather continues to learn and improve. Occasionally, teachers, doctors, or therapists have commented on how unusual it is for a child with her difficulties, at her age, still to be progressing. Sandra has sometimes said that she wishes she had known about the Feldenkrais Method when Heather was first diagnosed. I hope everyone who works with children will soon understand these ideas and ways to facilitate organic learning.

Creating Conditions for Learning

Organic learning begins even before birth and continues as long as one is alive. As one grows, with any weight gain or loss, with any illness or injury, through every process of aging, one experiences changes in self-image and way of functioning. When one is unaware, however, these changes can involve unwanted habits and behaviors that contribute to pains or problems.

With any approach to therapy or education, a percentage of people fail, including some who are capable, creative, and intelligent. Every failure, I believe, indicates that organic learning has been thwarted or frustrated in some way. Conventional notions commonly ignore or overlook the individual's active role in the healing process and credit treatments or techniques with bringing about cures. When effective, however, drugs or surgery, diets or exercises, prayers or psychotherapy or other interventions can be seen as ways to evoke, provoke, or encourage organic learning. Doctors, healers, teachers, therapists—the greatest of these, it seems to me, acknowledge that we heal ourselves.

191

All learning or healing involves organic learning. From my experience and from the experience of the thousands of people I have worked with, I know that each of us can and will heal and learn when possible. As a Feldenkrais practitioner, I view my role as creating favorable conditions for this to occur. To create those conditions, I need to be aware and prepared to learn, always respecting the unique needs and concerns of the person I am with, never assuming I already know what is right or needed. Thus, every Feldenkrais lesson is different. When working with someone individually, doing Functional Integration, one way I accomplish this is by using pads, pillows, or other props to vary the student's position each time.

When taught in person, not on prerecorded tapes or through written directions, Awareness Through Movement lessons are similarly customized for each person or group. Moshe created over one thousand lessons, with many variations of each, and in training new Feldenkrais Practitioners he encouraged us to be aware as we are teaching and to modify each lesson in appropriate ways. While individual Functional Integration and group Awareness Through Movement lessons appear quite different, both create conditions for organic learning in accordance with comprehensive functional insights into neurological development.

We learn most easily when relatively relaxed and comfortable and able to express curiosity freely. One way the Feldenkrais Method creates appropriate conditions is by doing lessons with people in their everyday clothes, neither undressing nor wearing special exercise outfits. When Moshe first began teaching individuals in the 1940s, he had his students undress for their lessons, but he saw that they put their habits and problems back on along with their clothes. In various ways, whether subtle or obvious, whatever one learns tends to be associated with the learning situation. Lessons are most functional when relatively familiar, as this facilitates transferring what one is learning to the everyday public domains in which the new choices and benefits of the lesson need to be available.

The year after I completed the Feldenkrais training, I met a man in his middle thirties who had been diagnosed with Friedrich's ataxia many years earlier. Joe had been active and healthy for his first eight years of life, began to have trouble with balance at the age of nine, could walk only with crutches when twelve, needed braces and crutches by the time he was sixteen, and had been in a wheelchair since he was nineteen. I worked with Joe for several months before I moved away from Santa Cruz, where he lived.

Friedrich's ataxia is described in the medical literature as a genetic, progressive, degenerative disorder of the cerebellum, an area at the base of the brain that coordinates all muscular activity. A neurologist I spoke with at the time gave me that information, photocopied from medical texts. What could I, or anyone, do about Friedrich's ataxia? Nothing, according to those experts.

When I was with Joe, however, I intentionally forgot those concepts and focused on his specific concerns and abilities. My role was to discover ways to create conditions in which he could become more aware and function more effectively. At the time we were learning together, Joe's speech was becoming difficult to understand and he was losing control of his right hand and arm, which had been dominant. Yet in spite of his difficulties, Joe lived alone, with an aide who visited only in the mornings and evenings, and he wanted to continue that arrangement. Due to the difficulty Joe had in transferring in and out of his motorized wheelchair, he remained in it during our lessons.

In every good Feldenkrais lesson, the practitioner acts with what Zen students call "Beginner's Mind," free of expectations, and I was truly a beginner, having never worked with, or even known, someone with difficulties like Joe's. In seeking to understand his experience, I practiced Awareness Through Movement and discovered ways to stiffen my shoulders and restrict my hand movements to only those he could do. I also found ways to thicken and distort my speech by contorting my neck, jaw, and tongue, and breathing irregularly. While I could move in those ways intentionally, Joe had no choice; he was doing the best he knew. For Joe to learn and improve, he first had to become aware of what he was doing.

When I was with Joe, I gently and precisely touched and moved him in ways that enabled him to sense which muscles were holding tighter than necessary. As he became more aware, those muscles relaxed, enabling us to discover ways for him to move more comfortably and effectively. One day, I walked in the front door of his home and saw him sitting at his kitchen table. Joe was holding the large metal mug he usually used, an empty bottle of his favorite fruit juice in front of him. As Joe slowly lifted the mug and drank, I noticed that he was holding the mug in his right hand, where before I had only seen him use the left in that way. He had been waiting, I understood instantly, to demonstrate that rediscovered ability. Joe finished drinking, lowered his mug, smacked his lips, and sighed. I simply smiled and said, "You really enjoyed that."

The last time I saw him, Joe described what the lessons had meant: "All my life, ever since I was a boy, each day I have been a little worse than the day before. Now, for the first time, I know the feeling of becoming a bit better."

Each of us can learn to reorganize and function more effectively, even those living with some neurological disorder or recovering from traumatic head injuries, in conditions that encourage organic learning and awareness.

Awareness

To appreciate how awareness heals, we need to understand what we mean by awareness. Yet neither dictionaries nor academic texts in psychology or philosophy provides clear, consistent definitions for either "awareness" or "consciousness," which some people use as a synonym for awareness. The terms "self-awareness" and "self-consciousness" compound this confusion, as does the fact that people sometimes speak of "higher consciousness," "higher awareness," or "conscious awareness."

Moshe was quite deliberate in his choice of words and sometimes commented on the challenge and importance of speaking carefully, since familiar words can lull us into complacency and assumptions that hinder constructive thinking. He maintained that there are four distinct states of existence—asleep, awake, conscious, and aware—and he thought of these experientially as constituting a series or hierarchy which involves the structure and functioning of the brain and nervous system. In my opinion, these ideas about the brain and experience provide clear, concrete, and useful ways to understand awareness.

We all know the difference between being asleep and being awake. Sleep involves withdrawal from time and space, and we sleep most deeply and restfully when we withdraw most completely. This withdrawal is especially evident in dreams, which are characterized by disruptions and distortions of time and space. We can also distinguish between being awake and being conscious. In casual speech, we do this when we use the term "conscious" to indicate that someone is focused or attentive, or when we describe someone who is daydreaming or disoriented as "unconscious." Every day, each of us experiences a brief period of being awake but not conscious—upon first awakening, when we think or ask, "Where am I?" You might recall times when you awoke in some unfamiliar setting, and the uncomfortable feeling of disorientation that sometimes accompanies such experiences. These examples suggest that orienting to space and in time is a fundamental function of consciousness.

In thinking about the brain, Moshe noted that sleep and wakefulness are coordinated by an area near the base of the brain called the reticular activating system. The reticular system, the limbic system, which regulates emotions and appetites, and areas that coordinate other basic biological functions are symmetrical and well-integrated, and they primarily utilize rapid serial connections between nerve fibers. In contrast, the cerebral cortex and forebrain are asymmetrical, evolved relatively recently, and operate mostly through parallel processing at approximately one-tenth the rate of older, deeper areas. The forebrain and cortex differentiate between and among actions and emotions by modulating the activity of the reticular system, limbic system, and related areas. Consciousness, in the view of most neuroscientists, depends on the forebrain and cortex, and Moshe thought that the complexity, asymmetry, and relative slowness of these areas make consciousness possible.

Questions about the evolution and unique characteristics of human consciousness concern many people. Meaningful answers, it seems to me, may be found in these insights into the brain's structure and the way consciousness involves orientation. With regard to the evolution of consciousness, the ability to orient and focus effectively and purposefully is essential for survival, and in Darwinian terms we can say that those who are best able to orient, focus, and achieve their goals are most likely to survive and reproduce. Human consciousness is characterized by language and symbolic capacities which enable us to orient or focus on events that are remote in time or space. We do this whenever we remember, imagine, or fantasize, and these capacities are essential for art, science, culture, and all that is uniquely human.

We are social beings, and our health and survival often depend on other people and our ability to communicate. We live in a world of words, a reality constructed through conversation and, once we learn to speak, inner dialogue. Language is linear and sequential, however, while experience is complex and multidimensional. Consciousness, when using language or focusing on particular goals, consequently tends to narrow our perceptions and exclude aspects of experience, limiting our ability to know ourselves or modify our behavior.

Awareness, as Moshe understood it, involves consciousness plus knowledge. To know what we are doing and learn, we need to be aware. Awareness links self and environment, inner experience with outer world, enabling us to be here, now, whole. The idea of a sequence from asleep to awake to conscious to aware suggested to Moshe that our capacity for awareness evolved even more recently than consciousness, involving the newest areas of the forebrain and a higher order of neurological complexity.

Here, respecting Moshe's insistence on making the abstract concrete, is a way to experience the distinction between consciousness and awareness: Imagine walking through your home and counting the number of windows. If you observe yourself carefully as you count, you will find that you make some small movement with your eyes, lips, tongue, or fingers as you note each window. You have been conscious while opening, closing, or looking through those windows in the past. Now, with this act of noticing and learning how you function, you are aware. You can do this again by naming the streets you cross during some familiar walk or drive, or by counting the number of letters in "Functional Integration". If you are sufficiently attentive, you will be able to identify subtle physical aspects of each of these "mental" acts.

Moshe understood that every act involves moving, sensing, feeling, and thinking. We are usually attentive to only one or two of these functions, however, while ignoring the others. With this experience of thinking about your home and counting the windows, you became aware of how you were simultaneously moving, and you did that by sensing your eyes, lips, tongue, or fingers. You were also feeling, and you are at this moment, even if you describe your feeling or emotional experience as normal or neutral. Generally, we are better able to think and sense and learn when relatively calm or emotionally neutral, since strong emotions overwhelm our capacity to make subtle distinctions. Immediately after any intense emotional experience, whether positive or negative, imagining and counting the windows in your home would be quite difficult. Probably, you would not be reading this book if you had just concluded a quarrel with your spouse, parent, or child. Your experience, I am sure, provides numerous examples of how every feeling or emotion involves changes in the way you move, sense, and think.

Whether you are aware or not, everything you do or know involves all of yourself. Yet each of us has learned, organically, to construct countless habits that streamline our actions and allow us to function without knowing what we are doing. Without habits, the simplest act would be impossible. For example, turning your head mobilizes dozens of muscles; alters sensory input from your eyes, ears, and kinesthetically; somehow expresses your feelings and intentions; and all of this simultaneously is organized by your nervous system without your awareness. Yet habits often become dysfunctional, as we all know. To learn and change, we need awareness so that, in an apparent paradox, we can function without awareness. Relative to habits, which are quick and powerful, acting with awareness is generally slow, subtle, tentative, inefficient. Amidst the stresses and demands of our busy lives, we often fail or forget to be aware. Also, habitual ways of speaking reinforce lack of awareness. This occurs whenever we discuss feelings or movements while ignoring sensing and thinking; describe hands, feet, head, or other "parts" of the body without considering the whole person; or talk of "self" while ignoring the fact that every self or individual always exists and acts in unique social and environmental contexts.

Did you actually perform those simple acts of sensing and observing yourself as you imagined and counted the windows in your home, named streets from a familiar walk or drive, or counted the letters in "Functional Integration"? If not, please pause for a moment and do so now. Immediately after doing that, notice how you are sitting and breathing, sensing and feeling and thinking. While reading, most of us are relatively unaware. Now, having performed these simple acts to evoke awareness, you may find that you are more aware of sensations, such as ambient light or sounds or the weight of your clothes. You may be breathing more easily or sitting more comfortably. You may feel more calm and peaceful. In addition, you may discover that you read, remember, and think more effectively.

These experiential and neurological insights into awareness are consistent with spiritual practices and psychological approaches, the way hypnosis, meditation, and similar techniques are described and used to quiet internal dialogue, enhance sensory acuity, and promote change. Social psychologist Ellen J. Langer, in her book, *Mindfulness* (Addison-Wesley, 1989), discusses research involving these practices and related experiences. What she describes as mindfulness applies to everything I am saying about awareness, and these terms are often used as synonyms in Buddhism and related traditions. In Langer's view, a mindful state of being includes several key qualities: "(1) creation of new categories; (2) openness to new information; and (3) awareness of more than one perspective" (p. 62). Langer also contrasts these qualities with the "mindlessness" that commonly characterizes everyday consciousness. In doing so, she reinforces and elaborates the distinction I am making between awareness and consciousness.

I like to picture consciousness as a spotlight that one can intentionally focus, but which always casts shadows and leaves some areas dark. This analogy suggests that "self-consciousness" involves focusing the spotlight on oneself, which is consistent with the way we commonly equate self-consciousness with either shyness or narcissism, since the shy person avoids what the narcissist craves, attention. When we clearly understand awareness as involving knowledge and relating oneself to one's environment, the term "self-awareness" becomes redundant. Statements that use this term, in my view, are equally meaningful when one either drops the prefix or substitutes "self-consciousness." While some people speak of "higher awareness" or "higher consciousness" when discussing intentional personal growth practices, "awareness," when truly understood, adequately describes the benefits of these activities. Since consciousness is often associated with language and awareness sometimes seems nonverbal, however, the term "conscious awareness" may be useful; it suggests an ability both to speak and to act in ways that respect one's wholeness, and, for me, this defines wisdom.

Awareness, to extend my analogy, is the light of the sun. You can see yourself and feel the warmth of the sun on your back while simultaneously looking out toward the horizon. Yet, just as a spotlight shining in your eyes blinds you to all else, awareness can be eclipsed if consciousness is too focused or purposeful. These analogies also remind us of the dangers of being unaware: we sometimes become sunburned when we sleep or play on the beach.

In varying ways and differing degrees, most pain and every problem indicates that one is or has been unaware. Awareness heals.

Health

You and I and all living organisms are self-maintaining, self-preserving, and self-reproducing, as described in the formal definitions used by biologists. Animals, insects, plants, and microorganisms die when they fail in any of these fundamental functions. As a scientist, Moshe recognized that a key indicator of health is the amount of stress which an organism can endure and from which an individual can recover. In enhancing your ability to recover from stress, you become healthier and more effectively self-healing.

In order to maintain, preserve, or reproduce ourselves, we need to move. For humans and all other animals, as distinct from plants and most microorganisms, the ability to move and explore the environment is fundamental to life and health. Those who lack or lose the desire and ability to do this survive only in extremely favorable conditions or through the care of others. Conversely, people who continue to be actively curious and interested in the world may confound a negative prognosis and recover from serious illnesses, sometimes unexpectedly or even miraculously.

When Moshe returned to Tel Aviv in 1950, he was asked to work with the prime minister, David Ben-Gurion, whose numerous health problems were not being helped by medical treatments. Ben-Gurion was 64 and living with such severe back pain and breathing problems that walking or simply arising from a chair was difficult. Yet Ben-Gurion was an exceptionally dynamic, powerful individual—a statesman who had studied law in several languages, who had labored for many years as a farmer, and had served as a soldier during the early settlement of Palestine.

In 1951, Moshe had not yet worked with many elder citizens, so he did not know if he could help Ben-Gurion. At their first meeting, Moshe began by sensing the movement in Ben-Gurion's head and neck. A mobile head is a biological necessity, required for perceiving the environment so that one can respond to threats or opportunities. If the head is not sufficiently mobile, muscles in the lower back, hip joints, and legs will continually overwork, breathing will be compromised, adequate relaxation will be unattainable, and there will be a general feeling of anxiety and stress. Ben-Gurion was experiencing all of these problems.

Yet Moshe was surprised to discover that Ben-Gurion's head moved perfectly within a small range. Recognizing that Ben-Gurion's genius extended to his physical functioning, Moshe knew he could help him. Later, Moshe asked Ben-Gurion to stand on a low stool and jump to the floor. Ben-Gurion, afraid of pain, could not do that, and he could not recall ever having done anything like it simply for his own enjoyment. Ben-Gurion had dedicated himself so totally to his dream of an independent state of Israel that he had profoundly neglected his own comfort and well-being.

For some time, Moshe saw Ben-Gurion regularly, even daily, and the two became extremely close friends. Throughout those years,

Ben-Gurion's health improved dramatically, and he began to delight in running up the stairs or through the hallways at the Knesset building, the meeting chamber of the Israeli Parliament. I do not know how they first conceived the idea, but at some point they agreed that Moshe would help Ben-Gurion learn to stand on his head. This was something Ben-Gurion wanted to do strictly for his own pleasure, with no other purpose. In October 1962, Ben-Gurion, then 76, was photographed standing on his head on the beach near his home in Tel Aviv. The picture was widely reprinted, appearing in *Parade* magazine in the United States.

Moshe taught the headstand in the second year of the Amherst training, but his way of doing that was quite different from any exercise or yoga technique. He wanted each movement to be completely effortless and reversible, meaning that at any point one could stop and smoothly change direction. We learned to lift our legs from the floor in many positions and return to the floor gently at different speeds, to twist and roll and fall in all directions, comfortably. An observer would not have known that what we were doing related to learning to stand on our heads, and for some time most of us students did not see that connection either. As the process continued, Moshe insisted that we not stand on our heads until doing so had become completely trivial. We learned to stand on our heads by recreating the way children learn to walk, playing and exploring comfortably. Moshe had followed the same process with Ben-Gurion.

Well before Ben-Gurion actually stood on his head, as Moshe told the story, a reporter had learned what they were doing and written about it in the newspaper. This provoked letters from leading doctors around the world urging Ben-Gurion to stop. The doctors insisted that, because Ben-Gurion was already in his seventies, standing on the head would cause a stroke and probably be fatal. When Ben-Gurion expressed doubts, Moshe responded, "Who's taking the greater risk, you or I? If you have a stroke, you'll be dead. I'll spend the rest of my life in jail or worse, scorned as the man who killed Ben-Gurion."

Ben-Gurion chose to continue. Moshe knew that the lengthy process they were following would gradually strengthen the blood vessels around the brain. Only the smallest would ever burst, without consequence, and those could be monitored by watching the tiny vessels in Ben-Gurion's eyes. Any increased redness in the eyes alerted them to slow the process and allow more time for recovery. In this way, Ben-Gurion's progress was continually regulated by his own physiology, as occurs with all truly organic learning.

I was in Israel with Moshe in the summer of 1983 and almost everyone I met knew his name because of his work with Ben-Gurion, who had lived to be 87 and remained healthy and politically active until the last few years of his life. Yet many people expressed surprise that I would consider Moshe so important as to travel from the United States to study with him. After returning to New York, where I was living at the time, I went to the public library one afternoon and looked through 25 biographies of Ben-Gurion. Most mentioned Ben-Gurion's lifelong poor health and the fact that he became increasingly robust and vigorous after age 65, while saying nothing about how this occurred. Three or four books told of some kind of treatment, without much explanation. Only one, *Prophet of Fire*, by Dan Kurzman (Simon and Schuster, 1983), described the lessons with Moshe, and how Ben-Gurion considered them so important that he scheduled cabinet meetings so as not to interfere.

I found that neglect quite interesting, but, upon reflection, not surprising. We have all been socialized to think of the body as a trivial machine, to ignore or deny the importance of our physical experience. How could Ben-Gurion's biographers appreciate the significance of his physical experience when they almost certainly had only limited awareness of their own ways of breathing, sitting, and walking?

When discussing his work with Ben-Gurion, Moshe described how the improvement in Ben-Gurion's physical capacities manifested in many ways: Ben-Gurion had always been intensely impatient and demanding, yet during the time they worked together he became increasingly tolerant, compassionate, peaceful. When you learn to be more aware and function more effectively, in any way, all aspects of your life improve and the world changes.

The Feldenkrais Method, as Moshe's work with Ben-Gurion and

my experiences with Joe and Heather illustrate, always images and orients toward ideal, healthy functioning. Consider how someone might ideally move: In any position or during any action, the skeleton supports the weight with every joint able to mobilize through its full range. Each muscle can contract completely as its opposite lengthens smoothly so that muscles everywhere have a balanced and relatively low tonus. A fully mobile neck and head enable the senses to monitor any changes in the environment. Breathing is free, with no inhibitions, even in difficult situations. All internal organs function harmoniously, with minimal energy. Any intention is enacted effortlessly, spontaneously.

Now observe yourself. How are you, at this moment, and habitually? How do you breathe, sit, walk? Do you experience any stiffness or discomfort, now or at other times? Are there activities which you enjoy but do not pursue because of some difficulty or disability?

Suppose you could take all your pains and problems and simply leave them behind, letting go of all your troubles, from the most severe to the utterly trivial. Just forget whatever may be bothering you: any stiffness in your back, tightness in your chest, or soreness in your feet; anger toward your mother, spouse, boss; fears, sadness, regrets. Imagine that, vividly. How would you feel? What would your life be like? Put this book down for a few moments to feel and think about how you would be if functioning more ideally.

You may want to walk around for a moment as if you really could leave all your troubles behind. Notice, or imagine, how you walk. How do you breathe? How does the world look to you? What are you aware of? What do you think about? Feeling like this, if you could do anything you want, what would you choose? Pause for a moment and consider these questions. Can you answer readily, or does this notion seem silly, unfamiliar, perhaps even somewhat uncomfortable?

To move and function ideally, to be so light and free and playful, might seem a wonderful fantasy. But if you could simply leave unwanted aspects or experiences behind, you would no longer be yourself. You learned to be who you are—a whole, integrated being. Any pains, problems, or disabilities are as essential to your self-image as your skills, talents, and abilities.

You can outgrow difficulties, however, just as a baby outgrows crawling. Babies fall many times as they learn to walk, and those falls are fundamental to the learning process. Similarly, any pains or problems you currently have may be like long, slow falls—vital steps in your learning. However you are, you can learn more comfortable and effective ways to function. Then you can move on to bigger challenges and more interesting problems, to further opportunities for growing and learning.

This is what the Feldenkrais Method really seeks: to create conditions that enable you to enhance your self-image, to help you grow and gain access to a greater range of possibilities. Not to treat or cure pains or problems, but to enable you to enjoy living as freely and fully as you choose.

As Moshe stated and demonstrated, to be healthy is to live for the realization of your avowed and unavowed dreams. Avowed dreams are the goals that we proclaim and pursue openly, dreams of fame and fortune, success and status, fancy cars and movie stars. These dreams typically reflect socialized expectations, yet we are social beings and benefit from expressing and pursuing these dreams, conditioned though they may be. Some people pursue these proudly shouted goals, however, while ignoring or denying dreams that speak only in shy, small voices. Unavowed dreams are like those each of us had as young children, dreams of flying and dancing and dissolving into joy, love, and wonder. Your unavowed dreams may be deep, subtle, and difficult to talk about, yet they still live. The true joy in life may be found in pursuing your unavowed dreams.

The healthiest individuals are living to pursue both avowed and unavowed dreams, whether they realize those dreams or not. As long as you are moving in that direction, by whatever indirect or circuitous route, your life will be filled with joy and meaning. Pain, suffering, and frustration are unavoidable; when you are true to your dreams, these become minor details in a rich tapestry, adding to the beauty of the pattern. Whatever may happen, you can recover and move forward to discover and realize new avowed and unavowed dreams.

Among the healthiest people I have known, some live in wheel-chairs or have been diagnosed with serious diseases, others have no money and few material comforts. Yet their eyes sparkle with passion and purpose. They laugh at times with no reason other than simple delight in being alive. I see that spirit, at least in brief flashes, in most people, and I feel tremendously sad at how we often deny or ignore our potential. Each of us can be more alive, creative, spontaneous, healthy.

However you are right now, whatever you may be doing, you can find ways to pursue your avowed and unavowed dreams. Your everyday experience can express the profound wisdom of your unique spirit. Here, now, you can begin to be more aware and healthy.

A World of Awareness

"Know thyself." Many people cite this phrase, from the oracle at Delphi in ancient Greece, as the key to wisdom. Yet few offer practical guidance on how to achieve self-knowledge.

The Feldenkrais Method is a way to learn. You can learn to relieve pain, recover from stress, improve athletic and artistic abilities, and enhance pleasure. You can learn, in the organic way of healthy children, to be more successful in everything you do. You can learn to realize your avowed and unavowed dreams.

Imagine a world which respects and truly values awareness and organic learning:

Back pain and most other musculoskeletal problems will be relatively rare and transitory. Currently, back pain is the most common reason people seek medical attention, affecting 80 percent of adults at some time in their lives.

Each of us will know how to learn, even in difficult circumstances, to function more comfortably and effectively. Stress, anxiety, and depression will be acknowledged as goads and guides for organic learning. This will enable us to save much of the 44 billion dollars currently estimated to be the direct and indirect costs of depression each year.

Children will learn more quickly and easily, in school and everywhere, with fewer academic or behavioral problems. Academic learning is commonly viewed as strictly mental, but sitting and reading are physical acts as well. As teachers learn to be more aware, they will know how to encourage children to breathe freely and sit comfortably, and this may help explain and resolve dyslexia and other learning disabilities.

Recovery from any sort of illness or injury will be accelerated as medical treatments work with the natural processes of organic learning. People diagnosed with stroke, cerebral palsy, multiple sclerosis, and other disorders will live rich, satisfying lives.

Athletes will set many new records. Actors, dancers, and musicians will achieve new levels of excellence. More important, we will all experience greater enjoyment and skill in whatever athletic and artistic activities we pursue.

Each of us will live longer and be healthier. Arthritis, heart dis-ease, and other illnesses that are currently viewed as degenerative, inevitable aspects of aging will be understood to involve years of inefficient habits. By integrating insights into organic learning with diet and exercise, we will discover ways to prevent or reverse many of these conditions.

These benefits may seem dramatic, yet they are readily achievable—and this is only the beginning of what we can expect. A world that respects and truly values awareness and organic learning will bring a renaissance in art, music, literature, science, psychology, philosophy, and all aspects of human experience. As we become more aware, we will also become more wise and compassionate, more respectful toward ourselves, toward each other, and toward our environment.

I want to live in that world and hope you will be there with me. Together, we can create it.

Appendix: For More Information

The Feldenkrais Guild

The Feldenkrais Guild is the professional association of Feldenkrais Method practitioners and teachers in the United States and Canada. You can contact them for names of Feldenkrais practitioners, a catalog of books and materials, and information about training programs.

The Guild is a nonprofit professional organization, concerned with increasing public awareness of the Feldenkrais Method, continuing education and certification of practitioners, protecting the quality and integrity of the Method, and supporting research into the Method's effectiveness. The Guild publishes the *Feldenkrais Journal,* a quarterly newsletter, and a directory of practitioners, which is updated annually. They welcome your inquiries.

The Feldenkrais Guild
P.O. Box 489
Albany, OR 97321-0143
800-775-2118
Fax: 541-926-0572
E-mail: feldngld@peak.org

Training in the Feldenkrais Method

Feldenkrais trainings provide unique environments for learning the theory and practice of the Feldenkrais Method. Through intensive Awareness Through Movement lessons, students learn about themselves and how they function, and this provides the foundation for learning to teach and practice Functional Integration. Theoretical insights and materials are integrated into these experiential processes, including anatomy, neurophysiology, biomechanics, cognitive science, human development, and related fields.

Trainings are held in many locations and follow various schedules, with each training taking $3\frac{1}{2}$ years, 40 days each year. This extended format enables and encourages students to integrate their Feldenkrais learning into their ongoing life activities. Each training is organized independently and accredited by the North American Training Accreditation Board, in association with the Feldenkrais Guild. Every training is supervised by an educational director and employs a minimum of four certified trainers during the course of the program. Certified assistant trainers maintain a low student/faculty ratio, insuring that students are adequately supported and exposed to a variety of teaching styles and perspectives. As part of the training process, each student receives periodic Functional Integration lessons from trainers and assistant trainers.

Upon successfully completing the training, students become eligible for certification and membership in the Feldenkrais Guild.

For information about upcoming trainings and related programs, please contact the Feldenkrais Guild.

The International Feldenkrais Federation

Feldenkrais guilds and associations operate in numerous countries and coordinate their activities through the International Feldenkrais Federation. Practitioners are active throughout Europe, Israel, Australia, New Zealand, Canada, Japan, and Latin America. Trainings are held in many countries.

For information about the International Feldenkrais Foundation and activities worldwide, please contact the Feldenkrais Guild.

Feldenkrais Resources

Feldenkrais Resources distributes books, tapes, and other materials on the Feldenkrais Method and related subjects, with some offerings not available from the Feldenkrais Guild. For a catalog, contact:

Feldenkrais Resources
830 Bancroft Way, #112
Berkeley, CA 94710
800-765-1907

Books by Dr. Moshe Feldenkrais

Moshe wrote for different audiences and purposes as his thinking and the Method evolved. Each of his books is uniquely valuable, yet every one has weaknesses and presents challenges. I list them here in the order in which I usually recommend them, with brief comments. All are available from the Feldenkrais Guild.

The Case of Nora (Frog Ltd, 1993)

Moshe originally told this story to a live audience, describing how he worked with a woman who had suffered a severe stroke. Nora was a well-educated woman in her sixties who spoke several languages. The stroke affected her coordination and left her unable to read and write, with a variety of related difficulties. Through recounting how he helped Nora, Moshe shares his insights into neurological development and general human functioning. This brief, inspiring book, first published in 1977, is Moshe's most readable.

Awareness Through Movement (HarperCollins, 1972)

This book uses 12 lessons to integrate concrete sensory-motor experience with fundamental insights into health, awareness, learning, self-image, and human nature. Moshe shows how learning to move with greater awareness and skill can improve all aspects of life, to benefit the individual, society, and humanity as a whole. The way the lessons are presented, however, makes them somewhat difficult to follow. Yet even if one never does the lessons, Moshe's philosophical perspectives make this book extremely valuable and thought-provoking.

The Elusive Obvious (Meta Publications, 1981)

In this, the last book Moshe wrote, he presents a general summary of his life and Method in a personal, anecdotal style. He describes many of the people he worked with over the years, both what he was doing and how he was learning in the process. Through many examples, he shows how each of us acts and thinks in habitual ways, that we are unaware of the extent to which habits inform our lives and self-images, and why attempts to change typically reinforce existing beliefs and behaviors.

The best way to resolve this dilemma, he shows, is to become more aware of concrete sensory-motor processes.

The Potent Self: A Guide to Spontaneity (HarperCollins, 1985)

Moshe wrote this book in the 1950s to show how his insights into movement and learning relate to psychological and social functioning. He was never satisfied with the text, however. After he died, the manuscript was reedited and published. This book presents many of Moshe's ideas quite usefully and powerfully.

The Master Moves (Meta Publications, 1984)

In 1979, Moshe taught a five-day workshop for a small group of people at the Mann Ranch in northern California. He was particularly pleased with that workshop, and this book is composed of the transcripts, which were edited by Carl Ginsburg, a Feldenkrais trainer, with assistance from Anat Baniel and Mark Reese, also Feldenkrais trainers, and Edna Rossenas. This book includes 12 lessons within a context of stories and theories that cover the full range of Moshe's thinking.

Body and Mature Behavior: A Study of Anxiety, Sex, Gravitation and Learning (International Universities Press, 1949, 1977)

In this scientific monograph, Moshe synthesized a vast body of research in neurophysiology, biomechanics, human development, and related fields. A great strength of this book, a key reason it continues to be valuable today, is that Moshe was able to escape the confines of any one discipline and apply diverse concepts to practical, everyday concerns. This book presents the key insights of the Feldenkrais Method in carefully detailed ways. I recommend this book to anyone who is not intimidated by scientific texts.

211

ACKNOWLEDGMENTS

Thanks, first, to my Feldenkrais friends and colleagues, especially Jerry Karzen, Allison Rapp, Larry Goldfarb, Anat Baniel, Jeff Haller, and Mia Segal. From Moshe, each of us learned in our own ways and developed our own "handwriting." Like any extended family, we have at times quarreled and criticized one another. Yet, somehow, we seem to have remained mostly true to our individual and shared dreams. I look forward to your comments and criticisms, and take full responsibility for my own interpretations and nonsense.

I also thank Mark Reese, Dennis Leri, Frank Wildman, Ruthy Alon, Marty Weiner, Carl Ginzburg, Yvan Joly, Donna Blank, Russell Delman, Alan Questel, Gaby Yaron, Chava Shelhav, Myriam Pfeffer, Yochanan Rywerant, and Kolman Korentayer. Many people have served and supported the Feldenkrais Guild through its struggles, and Bonnie Rich Humiston, Michael Purcell, and Nancy Schumacher deserve immense credit for their commitment and good humor. Thanks also to David Zemach-Bersin and Elizabeth Beringer for Feldenkrais Resources. Each of you, and countless others, has contributed to all that the Feldenkrais Method is becoming. In diverse ways, directly and indirectly, you have also enriched my life. Thanks.

The stories I tell in this book are all true and accurate to the best of my ability and recall. To all my students over the years, thanks—I hope you learned as much from our time together as I did.

This book, and learning to write generally, has been the most challenging and fulfilling task I have ever undertaken. A number of people expressed encouragement and assistance early in the process, when I most needed it, and I especially thank Judy Shafarman, Dale Lewis, Len Felder, Roslyn Targ, and Ted Berkman and Alan Rinzler at the Santa Barbara Writer's Conference.

I have appreciated my agent, Lynn Franklin, from our first conversation. Thanks, Lynn, for your enthusiasm, convictions, commitment, and gentle way of giving criticism. My editor, John Bell, seemed to appreciate my concerns and intentions so well that his suggestions often helped me discover what I wanted. I hope to write many more books, and feel quite blessed with this first experience. Thanks also to Mark Corsey, Lynne Reed, and everyone else at Addison-Wesley. Also to Ruth Linstromberg and Elizabeth Morales.

Over the years, many friends have been supportive, often in spite of my failure to express affection or appreciation. I particularly thank Carolyn Hawkins, J.W. Ballard, Bob Fitzgerald, Elisa Gottheil-Luciani, Catherine Sigal, Sandra McPherson, John Clausen, Nancy Gottlieb, James Hillman, Neil Marcus, Laurie Wilson, David Bermant and Susan Hopmans, Laura Lynn Schatz, Gail Kennedy, Don Shafarman, Linda Lyon, and Ilana Rubenfeld. Thanks also to Kay Izlar, Julius Dunworth, Julie McLeod, and everyone who keeps me dancing.

Finally, I offer especially heartfelt thanks to Jean Houston and Bob Masters for your early and continuing faith and encouragement, for introducing me to Moshe, and for your suggestions on revising this book and helping it be published. Jean has been a mentor and friend, a "beneficial presence" who has greatly enriched the lives of those who know her, and also has contributed to countless others who may never hear her name. One day, Jean, I hope you receive the acknowledgment you deserve. More than that, I wish for you a world in which people are individually and collectively rising toward a vision of the possible.

Years of thought and effort went into writing this book, and I know I have at times seemed aloof, distracted, impatient, arrogant, and otherwise unpleasant. Now that I have transformed this great and consuming intention into action, I hope to be a better friend to each and all of you. Thanks again.

INDEX

215